D0199055

BEYOND THE MAGIC BULLET

THE ANTI-CANCER COCKTAIL

A NEW APPROACH TO BEATING CANCER

BEYOND THE MAGIC BULLET

THE

A NEW APPROACH
TO BEATING CANCER

ANTI-CANCER
COCKTAIL

RAYMOND CHANG, MD

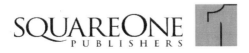

SQUAREONE
PUBLISHERS

The information and advice contained in this book are based upon the research and the personal and professional experiences of the author. They are not intended as a substitute for consulting with a health care professional. The publisher and author are not responsible for any adverse effects or consequences resulting from the use of any of the suggestions, preparations, or procedures discussed in this book. All matters pertaining to your physical health should be supervised by a health care professional. It is a sign of wisdom, not cowardice, to seek a second or third opinion.

EDITOR: Colleen Day
COVER DESIGNER: Jeannie Tudor
COVER PHOTOGRAPH: Getty Images, Inc.
TYPESETTER: Gary A. Rosenberg

Square One Publishers
115 Herricks Road
Garden City Park, NY 11040
(516) 535-2010 • (877) 900-BOOK
www.squareonepublishers.com

Library of Congress Cataloging-in-Publication Data
Chang, Raymond, 1957-
  Beyond the magic bullet : the anti-cancer cocktail / Raymond Chang.
     p. ; cm.
  Includes bibliographical references and index.
  ISBN-13: 978-0-7570-0232-8
  ISBN-10: 0-7570-0232-3
  I. Title.
  [DNLM: 1. Neoplasms--drug therapy. 2. Drug Therapy, Combination--methods. QZ 267]

  616.99'406--dc23
                        2011040831

Copyright © 2012 by Raymond Chang

All rights reserved. No part of this publication may be reproduced, stored in a retrieval system, or transmitted, in any form or by any means, electronic, mechanical, photocopying, recording, or otherwise, without the prior written permission of the publisher.

Printed in the United States of America

10   9   8   7   6   5   4   3

Contents

*"All men can see these tactics whereby I conquer,
but what none can see is the strategy
out of which victory is evolved."*

—SUN TZU

Acknowledgments

I would like to start by thanking Professor Mou Tsung-San, my philosophy mentor who, beginning nearly forty years ago, shaped my thinking, taught me to question conventionality, and encouraged me to think outside the box methodically and forcefully.

I offer my gratitude to the many doctors who influenced me throughout my medical and fellowship training. It was because of Dr. Bernard Shen, one of the most intelligent and multi-talented doctors I know, that I was able to hone the art of challenging conventional medical philosophy. I also thank Dr. Jeremiah Barondess, now President Emeritus of the New York Academy of Medicine and Professor Emeritus of Clinical Medicine at Weill Cornell Medical College, for further instilling in me the importance of rigorous medical thinking.

Additionally, I am indebted to those who were influential early on in my career at Memorial Sloan-Kettering Cancer Center. I am especially thankful to Dr. John Mendelssohn, who recruited me, and senior physicians Drs. Thomas Fahey and Larry Norton, along with many others, who served as role models and offered generous support during the decade I was there. I am also grateful to Dr. Sidney Winawer and the late Dr. William Fair, who pioneered and advocated an integrative approach to oncology when it was not yet popular, and who supported my endeavors to incorporate alternative medicine into conventional cancer care. I also thank my former Sloan-Kettering colleagues, including Drs. Yuman Fong, Nancy Kemeny, Phil Paty,

Paul Sabbatini, Stephen Veach, and many others, for their continued support.

During my fifteen years in private practice, I have received the gracious support of many open-minded oncologists and physicians, including Drs. Abraham Chachoua, Anna Gattani, Roger Granet, Stuart Leitner, Anne Moore, George Raptis, Lynn Ratner, Max Sung, Linda Vahdat, and Marisa Weiss. I am greatly appreciative of their kind willingness to share their cases with me. I would also like to thank my many colleagues in complementary and alternative medicine for their support and friendship: Drs. Benjamin Kligler, Roberta Lee, and Woodson Merrell of the Beth Israel Continuum Center for Complementary and Alternative Medicine; Dr. Keith Block of the Block Center for Integrative Care; Dr. James Gordon of The Center for Mind-Body Medicine; Dr. Mark Renneker of San Francisco; Dr. Jeffrey White of the National Cancer Institute; Dr. Shaw Chen of the Food and Drug Administration; Elenas Ladas of Columbia University; and Dr. Fredi Kronenberg from the former Rosenthal Center at Columbia Presbyterian Medical Center. Ralph Moss—a friend, mentor, and constant source of inspiration—deserves special mention; he was among the first to challenge conventional cancer treatments, and he continues to be one of the leading sources of knowledge on unconventional treatments, both in the United States and abroad. Ken Schueler, cancer patient advocate par excellence, also deserves my special thanks for sharing his patients, ideas, and enthusiasm for better treatments.

Of course, I am indebted to Dr. David Ho and his inspiring discovery of cocktail therapy for HIV, which transformed treatment for the once-deadly disease. I am personally grateful to Dr. Benjamin Williams, not only for taking the time to write the Foreword to this book, but also for advancing cocktail therapy for cancer, using himself as an example.

I would be remiss if I did not mention my father and mother, who raised me to think independently and tolerated my childhood tendency to not always follow rules. I also owe a tremendous amount to the love of my family, Grace in particular, who were patient with me as I took time away from them in order to write this book.

For the concept of the cocktail therapy discussed in this book, I perhaps owe more to my patients than any colleague, teacher, book, journal, seminar, or course. They believed in my work, entrusted me with their lives, and allowed me to do what I thought was best for them. They also allowed me to share in their karma, challenged me with their illness and pain, and served as my eyes and ears by bringing new and different treatments to my attention. It is with them, and only because of them, that I developed and fine-tuned my theoretical framework for a cocktailed approach to cancer.

For years, I had been planning to summarize my ideas for a different approach to cancer treatment, but wanted to wait until retirement so as to have more time and free myself from any professional controversy that might ensue. But two years ago, over a cup of coffee in a diner, my publisher, Rudy Shur, convinced me to take up the challenge now instead. Rudy was especially kind in giving me extra latitude to express myself in my own words and work at my own pace. He also provided me with numerous suggestions for communicating this difficult subject to the public more effectively. This book is much indebted to him. Finally, I would like to thank my forever patient editor, Colleen Day, who has been indispensable from day one, for combing through the manuscript and making many useful changes and suggestions.

Foreword

Although the past twenty years have seen considerable progress in the treatment of some cancers, others have remained intractable. Among the worst are pancreatic cancer, metastatic melanoma, and glioblastoma multiforme, a type of brain cancer that I myself was diagnosed with over sixteen years ago. These are still considered death sentences, as are many other cancers once they have spread.

Why some forms of cancer are more treatable than others is not well understood. Cancers vary in the number of their genetic mutations, with the presumption that those with many mutations will make the task of finding effective treatments more difficult. Even when some aberrant growth pathways can be inhibited or eliminated, others remain and become amplified by the process of evolutionary selection. As a result, most oncologists agree that single-agent treatments are unlikely to be successful. This opinion is buttressed by the recognition that some forms of cancer treatment have been revolutionized by the development of treatment cocktails. For cancers such as childhood leukemia, cocktail therapy has been far more effective than treatments based on individual agents.

Unfortunately, current policy regulating the development of new treatments has largely been based on a single-treatment mentality. Initial clinical trials almost never involve combinations of treatments, which occur only when the individual single agents have shown some degree of effectiveness. This policy thwarts effective cancer treatment in several ways. The most obvious is that it greatly slows the development of the treatment cocktails that will be necessary for cancer treatment to be successful. It also creates false negatives, as drugs that can be effective components of a treatment cocktail may not be effective as single agents. It may also make the eventual use of a treatment cocktail less effective, as the development of resistance to treatment agents presented individually causes the cocktails that contain these agents as components to be less effective.

Yet, patients, with the help of their oncologists, need not settle for the snail's pace of the development of new treatments. We now know that many medications developed for various medical conditions other than cancer possess anti-cancer properties. Because they are off-patent, many of these drugs are never tested in conventional cancer clinical trials so that the revenue generated by their anti-cancer usage does not justify the enormous cost of conducting the trials. Moreover, many foods and dietary supplements also have significant anti-cancer properties. Thus, as Dr. Chang proposes in this book, we may not need newer and better drugs for cancer, but rather a better way of using what we already have. Based on my own experience and that of patients whom I have advised, I believe that existing knowledge about the anti-cancer properties of non-standard treatment agents may be enough for the development of effective treatment cocktails *now,* not some distant time in the future.

The great majority of patients who have sought to use treatment cocktails have received minimal cooperation from their oncologists. One reason for this is that medical dogma requires treatments to pass the test of randomized clinical trials before they can be used as treatments outside of clinical trials. In actuality, there is no absolute legal basis for this restriction; any physician can legally prescribe any FDA-approved drug for any purpose, not just for the purpose for which the drug was initially approved. However, doctors tend to be conservative and in fear of unnecessary liability when they do not follow standards of practice. Furthermore, insurance companies often do not pay for off-label treatments.

When diseases have been persistently intractable to the best standard of care, as defined by conventional medical standards, common sense dictates that we enlist all possible treatment resources, not just those that have passed the test of trials. Other forms of evidence can also be convincing, and randomized clinical trials themselves have their own problems of interpretation. Phase II clinical trials, which are not usually randomized, contain a rich source of information, as do experimental results from animal models, especially with respect to possible synergies between treatment agents.

Given that oncologists, in general, have tacitly accepted the principle that treatment cocktails may be necessary for effective treatment of many types of cancer, what explains the opposition to their use? There is, of course, no opposition after an effective cocktail has been identified in well-controlled clinical trials. However, their preliminary development will have highly variable components, depending on the interpretation of the existing evidence regarding synergy among the individual components. Therefore, doctors who use cocktail treatments in their clinical practice do so under the cloud of being unscientific and at risk of being labeled proponents of alternative medicine, which carries a significant stigma among the conventional medicine camp. But such concerns say more about maintaining hegemony by the professional guild than concern for patient welfare. This is especially true when dealing with diseases for which conventional medicine concedes that it offers no effective treatments.

When I was diagnosed with glioblastoma multiforme sixteen years ago, conventional treatment offered no hope that I could survive my disease. But it seemed obvious to me that the HIV cocktail offered a model for how to proceed. My approach was thus to identify those treatment agents that had been shown to have some degree of efficacy for my disease and combine as many as possible. Yet I could follow this path only by surmounting the obstacles imposed by my physicians. What I needed then, and what continues to be needed by patients today, is a physician like Dr. Chang, who has a broad knowledge of different treatment modalities and appreciates the importance of treatment combinations.

Dr. Chang, as he humbly emphasizes, did not invent the idea of cocktail therapy for cancer treatment, but he has taken an important first step towards scientifically justifying its use. In *Beyond the Magic Bullet,* he eloquently explains why the cocktail approach is superior to the linear, or "one-drug-at-a-time," strategy that dominates present cancer care. Dr. Chang's book will hopefully advance the discussion of the cocktail strategy so that it can one day become a standard practice in cancer therapy and ease the burden of patients seeking effective treatment.

Ben Williams, PhD
Professor Emeritus of Psychology,
University of California at San Diego
Author of *Surviving "Terminal" Cancer: Clinical Trials, Drug Cocktails, and Other Treatments Your Oncologist Won't Tell You About*

Introduction

Since the National Cancer Act declared "war" on the disease in 1971, cancer has been likened to an enemy that must be fought and defeated. Over the last several decades, billions of dollars have been poured into stopping cancer in its tracks and, today, there is a wealth of information about cancer biology and hundreds of cancer therapies. Yet, a cure has yet to be found. As the title of a 2008 *Newsweek* article summed it up, "We fought cancer . . . and cancer won." This predicament has left many scientists and doctors wondering whether the time has come to rethink how the war on cancer should be carried out. Like any war, the war against cancer cannot be won with weapons and firepower alone; an effective strategy is also essential. And this may be the key that is missing.

The study of cancer is a science, but the treatment of cancer involves both science and strategy. While the science may be accurate, the dominant strategy for treating the disease has been largely influenced by medicine's past success against infectious disease. The effectiveness of antibiotics in killing germs and curing infections shaped the way that doctors approached disease, including cancer, which was initially viewed as a foreign entity that invaded the body. Many believed that curing cancer depended on finding the right medicine to kill the cancer "bug." And it was from this point of view that the hunt for a "magic bullet," or single-solution cure, was born. In other words, it was assumed that cancer was like a vault with a single lock, and with only one key that could open it. If only the right key was found, then, like magic, the vault could be unlocked. The possibility that cancer had several "locks," or even a combination lock, was not widely considered, nor was the idea that patients could have different sets of locks unique to their individual cancers. Instead, the simple "hit or miss" strategy persisted and dominated cancer treatment philosophy.

Today, however, there is a growing appreciation of the complex biology of the phenomenon known as cancer. As single-agent therapies continue to prove insufficient, it has become apparent that a single "key," or magic bullet cure, may simply not exist for most cancers. Rather, the simultaneous use of multiple "bullets" to target cancer's multiple dimensions and pathways may be a more appropriate strategy. This combination, or "cocktail," strategy is neither new nor unique, though it has not been commonly practiced in Western medicine. In contrast, the strategy has been employed in Traditional Chinese Medicine (TCM) for thousands of years in the form of herbal "cocktail" formulas, acupuncture, and other multidimensional treatment methods.

A turning point for Western medicine came in 1994 when Dr. David Ho, in what he referred to as a "Eureka moment," applied the cocktail strategy to HIV therapy and, in turn, revolutionized treatment for the virus.[1] Furthermore, in 1995, Dr. Ben Williams adopted this strategy to fight a deadly brain tumor, using a cocktail of conventional and alternative therapies.[2] Williams' "anti-cancer cocktail" was successful, and he has become cancer-free. These examples show that cocktail therapy is a viable strategy that has proven successful in many cases. Now, it is necessary to establish a logical basis for using cocktail therapy to treat malignant cancers of any type and at any stage. That is what this book hopes to achieve.

Divided into two parts, *Beyond the Magic Bullet* covers cocktail therapy both in theory and in practice. Part 1, "The Biology and Treatment of Cancer," makes the case for cocktail therapy as a strategy that takes the biological complexity of cancer into full account. Chapter 1 provides an introduction to this complex biology, explaining the numerous ways in which cancer may arise and spread throughout the body. Conventional treatments for the disease are outlined in Chapter 2, including classical methods like chemotherapy as well as modern targeted therapies. Chapter 3 takes a look at the competing medical philosophies underlying conventional cancer treatment and cocktail therapy, the pros and cons of which are carefully weighed in Chapter 4. Finally, in Chapters 5 and 6, the actual practice of cocktail therapy is examined in more detail. Here, you will learn about the various "ingredients"—vitamins, herbs, supplements, pharmaceutical drugs, diets, spiritual activities, and more—that may comprise an anti-cancer cocktail. You will also become familiar with the treatment process, from choosing a doctor to the step-by-step implementation of therapy. This information will help you ensure the best possible cancer care.

Part 2 is split into two sections that list various pharmaceutical drugs and supplements that may be effective for treating and/or preventing cancer. When combined with conventional therapies, these agents may increase the odds of treatment success and survival. These lists are neither comprehensive nor intended to replace the expert advice of a healthcare professional. Still, they can serve as a valuable resource when considering cancer treatment options. You can then turn to the Appendices and read three case studies demonstrating how anti-cancer cocktails have been safely and successfully implemented for three actual cancer patients. These cases highlight the potential of cocktail therapy to change how we approach the treatment of cancer.

Beyond the Magic Bullet is not a self-treatment manual or a recipe book for cancer therapy, but rather a blueprint for a superior treatment strategy. As cancer researchers continue to look for more effective treatments, cocktail therapy may be better able to slow down, stop, and even reverse the disease in the meantime. This book was written in hopes of giving patients an alternative by providing vital information to share and discuss with their physicians. If you or someone you love is affected by cancer, *Beyond the Magic Bullet* can be the "map" that assists you in navigating this complex and difficult disease.

I believe that cancer is curable, perhaps in our lifetime. I have full faith in the good work that my colleagues are doing today to discover better cancer treatments for tomorrow. At the same time, I believe that a radically different strategy is needed, because cancer simply cannot wait for clinical trials to be completed or for drugs and other therapies to be approved. Careful re-strategizing with our existing arsenal of treatments may produce dramatically improved results *now*. The time has come to think beyond the magic bullet.

PART 1

The Biology and Treatment of Cancer

1

The Biology of Cancer

With the wide range of treatments at hand today, we should be able to revolutionize our treatment of cancer. The limitations of current cancer therapy may not be due to a lack of understanding of how the disease works or a lack of effective treatments, but rather a failure to implement an optimal treatment strategy *despite* what we know and have. The limitations of the conventional cancer treatments—surgery, chemotherapy, radiation, and newer targeted therapies—may largely result from the one-dimensional and simplistic strategy that is usually followed to the exclusion of other approaches. But to appreciate the possibility of a new cancer treatment strategy, we must first understand the complex and diverse nature of the disease, which is often overlooked, as well as the limitations of the standard treatments used in conventional medicine. This understanding will provide a rational basis for using a new approach that could potentially revolutionize cancer therapy.

THE COMPLEXITY OF CANCER

To devise a better treatment strategy for cancer, it is essential to understand the complexity of cancer biology. The first question we must ask is, "What is cancer?" According to the National Cancer Institute (NCI), cancer can be defined simply as "diseases in which abnormal cells divide without control and are able to invade other tissues." But if uncontrolled growth is all there is to cancer, effective treatments would need only stop or reduce the growth in the same way that antibiotics kill bacteria. Obviously, cancer has proven itself to be not so simple a condition, as we have not yet invented or found an antibiotic capable of killing the cancer "germ."

Cancer is like the multi-headed hydra. It involves not only complex genetic and molecular pathways that control cell growth, but also dynamic interactions between cells and their surrounding tissue environment. Cancer's deadliness is due to its inability to stop multiplying, its tendency to spread and recur, and its capacity to build resistance to treatment. An insightful description of the disease was recently put forth by a group of scientists: "Cancer cannot be simply understood as individual mutations. The effect of a mutation often depends on the context of other mutations within the same cell, the context of other mutant cells within the same tumor, and the context of . . . the environment of the tumor and the patient."[1] Therefore, in order to better understand the nature of this deadly disease, let's begin by looking at its initiation and its progression—two aspects of cancer that reveal its complexity and diversity.

The Initiation of Cancer

The word *cancer* is a general descriptive term that encompasses more than 100 distinct abnormal conditions in the human body. Cancer is complex in its forms and its formation, or *initiation*—the term used to describe the complexities that bring about cancer and how the disease manifests in the body. Cancer can arise in any organ and affect various types of cells, such as blood cells, germ cells, epithelial or lining cells, glandular cells, and nerve cells. Sometimes, cancer may affect more than one type of cell within the same organ. Some forms of cancer have a hormonal component (breast and prostate cancer) or a hereditary component (breast cancer, ovarian cancer, and melanoma). The initiation of cancer can also be related to gender or age; there are cancers that occur more frequently in women than men and vice versa, and cancers that affect children more than adults. For example, children are more frequently diagnosed with certain forms of leukemia as well as cancers of the central nervous system, such as medulloblastoma and neuroblastoma.

In addition, cancer's initiation may be linked to ethnicity, geography, or lifestyle, as well as exposure to sunlight, chemicals, parasites, viruses, and certain bacteria. For instance, nasopharyngeal cancer is more common among the Chinese population, while Burkitt's lymphoma occurs most frequently among people from equatorial Africa. Lifestyle factors can also play a role in cancer development, as smoking is a known risk factor for lung cancer, and shift work has been associated with breast cancer risk. Moreover, excessive exposure to sunlight is correlated with skin cancer, and contact with chemicals such as aflatoxin, benzene, and asbestos may cause liver cancer, leukemia, and mesothelioma, respectively. There are also microbes that can initiate the disease, like the parasite *Clonorchis sinensis* (gallbladder cancer), the bacterium *Helicobacter pylori* (stomach cancer), and a number of viruses, including hepatitis B and C (liver cancer), the Epstein-Barr virus (nasopharyngeal cancer and some lymphomas), and the human papillomavirus (cervical cancer). Still, most cancers have unspecified causes or are caused by a multiplicity of factors and further affected by genetics, diet, environment, and even emotions.

The Progression of Cancer

The *progression* of cancer, which refers to its growth and proliferation, as well as the various ways in which it evades medical intervention, is at least as complicated and diverse as its initiation. Some cancers are fairly slow-growing, taking their toll over the course of a decade or more, while other types are aggressive, tearing through a life in a matter of months. Inexplicably, some cancers even shrink on their own. (Unfortunately, most do not.)

Cancer generally grows in a series of steps. These steps range from *hyperplasia*, a condition in which a normal-looking cell cannot stop multiplying; to *dysplasia*, when cells appear to have abnormalities, mutations, or atypical structural changes within them; to *anaplasia*, in which cells completely lose properly functioning structures. All of these steps reflect the cells' increasing loss of self-control, or what is called *uncontrolled cell division*. The final phase involves wild and unbridled cell growth.

The uncontrolled cell growth that characterizes cancer is a result of disturbances within the cell's growth cycle, which may be caused by genetic changes or mutations. For example, when *proto-oncogenes,* which normally control cell signals, mutate to become *oncogenes,* cell growth switches into overdrive. Additionally, defects can occur in *tumor suppressor genes* (or anti-oncogenes), which act as brakes to cell growth, as well as genes that normally have a repair function, in turn leading to cellular disrepair. As if this wasn't complex enough, disruptions in the cellular growth cycle can also be connected to an imbalance of proteins, such as *cyclin-dependent kinases* (CDKs), which were discovered and characterized in the 1990s. The synchronization of a cell's growth cycle depends on a balanced amount of these proteins, which is disturbed in most cancers. (See Figure 1.1 on page 11.) In sum, cancer can be viewed as a genetic malfunction at the most basic DNA level, or as a dysfunction at a higher level of cellular activity—cell signaling, programming, and other regulatory processes.

A recent study published in *Science* provides a glimpse of the complexity with which we are dealing. An international research team sequenced more than 20,000 genes in cells from twenty-four patients with advanced cancer and found that a typical case of cancer involves an average of sixty-three genetic mutations involving twelve abnormal cellular pathways. Delving further into this complexity, a new field of biology called *epigenetics* has highlighted the importance of not only mutations and defects at the DNA level, but also the "switching on and off" of otherwise normal genes, an abnormal process that is affected by a web of other processes. This phenomenon can be likened to identical twins: Their genes may be completely identical, but there are differences between the two in part because some genes that are active in one twin may not be active in the other. The "turning on" of cancer-promoting genes and the "turning off" of cancer-suppressing genes plays a key role in the development of cancer, from its initiation to its progression.

There are other important aspects of cancer progression beyond simple cell growth, including the ability of cancer cells to invade tissue, spread to distant sites in the body, build up resistance to treatment agents, and escape the body's immunological detection. Cancer cells even have the uncanny ability to circumvent therapies directed

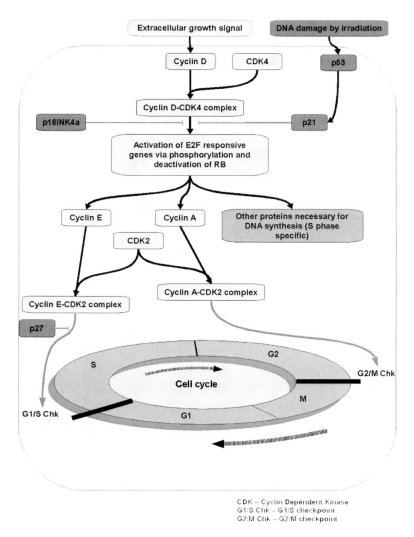

FIGURE 1.1. REGULATION OF CELL GROWTH CYCLE. A simplified representation of some of the molecular and genetic control mechanisms that affect the growth of a cell, each of which acts as a potential target for cancer therapy.

at them. Indeed, *multidrug resistance* (MDR) is a major hindrance to effective cancer treatment. MDR occurs in cancer cells in which the MDR-1 gene is overexpressed, as this gene is responsible for coding *P-glycoprotein* (P-gp). This substance, which is overproduced in such cancer cells, acts as a "pump" to remove anti-cancer drugs directed at the cell.

All of this information is not intended to leave your head spinning, but rather illustrate the complexity of cancer. This disease involves the interaction of cancer cells and their genetic and subcellular functions, the surrounding tissue environment, and the immune system. In recent years, scientists have also learned that the cancer's immediate environment—its blood and nutrient supply, acidity and oxygen levels, and balance of cellular signals called *cytokines*—also intimately affects the progression of the disease. In other words, cancer is not a stand-alone phenomenon.

THE NATURE OF THE BEAST

Hardly half a century ago, scientists understood cancer simply as unrestrained cell growth. Yet as Fabio Grizzi, a researcher at the Instituto Clinico Humanitas in Milan, has observed, medical scientists have been looking for simplicity only to find more complexity.[2] As such, the scientific community may be finally awakening to the enormous difficulty of the challenge we are facing.

In January 2004, a fierce snowstorm crippled much of the Washington, DC area, but it did not stop more than seventy doctors and researchers from traveling to the National Cancer Institute for a landmark meeting about its newly formed Integrative Cancer Biology Program (ICBP). Recognizing the inadequacy with which cancer biology had been researched and understood in the past, the program was intended to launch initiatives focusing on the complexity of cancer, with the overall goal of promoting the disease as a complicated biological system.

Dr. Dinah Singer, Director of the NCI Division of Cancer Biology, put it like this: "We now appreciate that cancer is a disease of genes and we understand the regulation and function of a huge number of these genes. . . . We have [a] detailed understanding of how proteins interact, both structurally and functionally, in regulatory, signaling, and metabolic pathways. What we are lacking is a systematic approach to integrate various kinds of data and processes. . . where we can analyze the complex biological systems that are cancer."[3] In other words, although we may understand the individual parts and underlying mechanisms of cancer, we have not been able to completely grasp the whole. We can see the trees, but not the forest.

A comprehensive basis for understanding the intricate biological interplay that constitutes cancer is the prelude to a radical rethinking of a better treatment strategy for the disease. Where does this understanding leave us with the direction of treatment? It is obvious that a simple condition can be treated simply, as a strep throat can be healed with penicillin. But a disease like cancer should not—and cannot—be treated using the same simplistic strategy of applying one drug at a time, one punch after another. Now that we know how many heads this "hydra" called cancer has, it is clear that we need not only new and improved medicine, but also a new and improved strategy that reflects and addresses the complexity of the disease.

CANCER BIOLOGY'S IMPLICATIONS FOR A NEW STRATEGY

Over a decade ago, scientists thought that exhaustively identifying, studying, and describing the parts, processes, signals, and pathways of cell growth would lead to innovations in cancer treatment. Robert Weinberg, a professor of biology at the Massachusetts Institute of Technology who identified the first oncogene and suppressor gene, predicted that "a new set of talents will be brought to bear on the cancer problem. Mathematicians with expertise in analyzing complex multicomponent systems will explain how the minicomputers inside cells actually function. . . . With increasingly detailed information on the metabolism of normal and cancerous cells, it will become possible to design highly selective drugs that strike cancer cell targets."[4] In reality, however, effective cancer treatment will likely involve more than understanding the details of cell growth. As scientists have uncovered the underlying genetics of both normal and cancerous cells, the mechanisms and deficiencies of the immune system, and the pathways by which cancer cells spread and invade other tissues, they are increasingly appreciative of how complicated a disease cancer truly is. Figure 1.2 (see page 14), which illustrates a typical cancer cell pathway, provides a glimpse of the degree of complexity involved. As Dr. Bert Vogelstein of Johns Hopkins University succinctly put it in a recent interview, "Cancer is very complex—more complex than we had believed."[5]

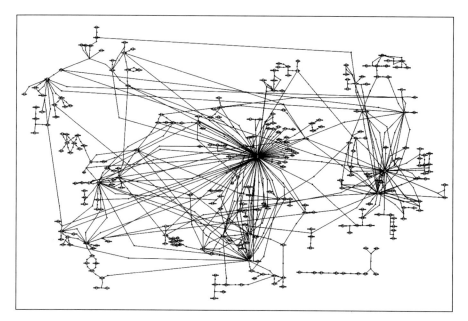

FIGURE 1.2. CANCER CELL MAP. One of many possible complex genetic pathways of a cancer cell. This one involves a specific growth signal known as the epidermal growth factor (EGF) of the EGF receptor (EGFR) family. This pathway is involved in regulating a number of importaznt processes, including cell proliferation, and is the target of some modern cancer therapies.

CONCLUSION

In order to set the stage and provide a rationale for a better treatment strategy, we must start by emphasizing—and, more importantly, understanding—the complexity of cancer. It would be naive to imagine a complex problem to be solvable in simplistic terms. Current treatment methods such as surgery, chemotherapy, radiation, and simple drug regimens applied one after another reflect such naivety. Before presenting a new strategy for cancer based on a deeper biological understanding of the disease, we will first go over these conventional medical treatments and their shortcomings. The next two chapters provide a picture of where we stand today in terms of cancer treatment.

2

Conventional Cancer Treatments

As demonstrated by recent advances in cancer research, the modern era is seemingly one of limitless information and technological advances. We know more about the complexity of cancer than ever before, including how it starts, behaves, and spreads throughout the body. However, our current ability to treat the disease pales in comparison to the knowledge we have about it. The classical treatments that form the backbone of current cancer therapy—surgery, chemotherapy, radiation, and hormone therapy—have been employed for a long time but, in many instances, remain quite limited in their ability to cure or even curb the disease. And although recent years have seen many medical breakthroughs and more cutting-edge treatments, novel therapies are generally used only when the standard treatments fail.

Simply put, the current strategy and standards for treating cancer are inadequate. As a result, survival rates for many cancers—such as brain, colorectal, lung, and pancreatic cancer—have not significantly improved over the last thirty years. This chapter reviews the conventional treatment methods, both classical and modern, that comprise cancer therapy today and explains why they are insufficient.

CLASSICAL CANCER TREATMENTS

Up until the turn of the twenty-first century, there were few treatment options for a person diagnosed with cancer. With the exception of hormone therapy, cancer treatment was focused largely on the annihilation of cancer cells. The cancer was removed surgically (in the form of a tumor), eliminated with drugs and chemicals via chemotherapy, or destroyed with radiation. These four methods—surgery, radiation, chemotherapy, and hormone therapy—continue to serve as the mainstay of cancer treatment. Despite the success of these treatments for some localized and early-stage cancers, as well as less common cancers such as testicular cancer and some forms of leukemia and lymphoma, such treatments cannot effect a cure for the majority of adult cancers. Worse is the fact that some of them, particularly radiation and chemotherapy, are toxic and cause undesirable side effects, in turn placing limits on how long and intensely they can be used. This section takes a closer look at each of these treatments and their limitations.

Surgery

The physical removal of tumors and tumor tissue with surgery is a conventional cancer treatment that has been employed since ancient times. The earliest surgery on record took place in 1500 BC in Egypt and involved the cauterizing (burning out) of breast tumors with an instrument known as a fire drill. Approximately 600 years later, the prominent Roman physician Galen advocated the cauterization of tumors, convinced that it was an effective way to treat and even cure cancer. By the seventh century, physicians such as Paul of Aegina of the Byzantine Empire, began to favor the physical removal of tumors over cauterization. But it was not until the nineteenth century that surgery was established as the mainstay of cancer therapy. With the emergence of major surgical advances such as general anesthesia, renowned doctors like Freund, Billroth, Handley, and Halsted were able to perform landmark operations that forever changed how cancer was approached and treated.

Today, there are a number of surgeries for fighting and eliminating cancer. The area of the body affected and the goal of treatment determines the type of surgery that will be performed. In addition to *curative surgery,* which removes the cancer in its entirety to cure the patient, there is also *debulking surgery* to reduce the cancer in size and render it more treatable through other methods like chemotherapy and radiation. *Preventive surgery* is used to remove an organ at risk for developing cancer, *diagnostic surgery* (or *staging surgery*) is performed to identify the nature and extent of cancer in a patient, and *palliative surgery* reduces any pain or discomfort experienced as a result of the disease. Moreover, there are now technologically advanced forms of surgery that allow access to parts of the body that are difficult to reach and often result in better outcomes. These include *laser surgery, cryosurgery, laparoscopic surgery, robotic surgery,* and *microscopically controlled surgery.* (See the inset on page 20.) In many cancer cases, surgery still offers the best chance for survival—especially for early-stage cancer—and is a key aspect of cancer management.

Radiation

Radiation is another classical mechanism for treating cancer. Even low levels of radiation are *cytotoxic*—that is, able to kill cells, especially rapidly dividing cancer cells. The origin of radiation is the x-ray, a form of electromagnetic radiation discovered by the German physicist Wilhelm Roentgen in 1895. This famous breakthrough inspired Emil Grubbe, a medical student in Chicago, to test the effectiveness of radiation for breast cancer therapy the following year. Grubbe's experiment was successful, and by the early twentieth century, radiation therapy was a routine medical practice for cancer treatment. Today, it is estimated that 60 percent of cancer cases, from solid tumors to lymphoma, are treated with radiation.

However, radiation therapy presented one major challenge: It tended to damage healthy tissue and properly functioning cells in the process of destroying harmful cancer cells. But as technology has advanced, medical scientists have found more efficient ways to target tumors while sparing the surrounding healthy tissue. New medical equipment with computer-assisted tracking and controls has enabled targeted radiation techniques such as *multidimensional conformal therapy, intensity-modulated radiation therapy* (IMRT), *stereotactic radiosurgery* (CyberKnife, Gamma Knife), *proton beam radiation therapy,* and *radioimmunotherapy.* (See the inset on page 20.)

Another specialized method of radiation is *brachytherapy,* which is the implantation of a radioactive source, such as pellets, seeds, or catheters, in or near the cancerous tissue. This is a preferred alternative to shooting external beams of radiation at cancer cells because it minimizes damage to surrounding tissues. In some circumstances, a radioactive substance may be taken orally or injected directly into the bloodstream. This type of treatment is called *systemic radiation therapy,* and it can be curative in early-stage cancers of the prostate and thyroid, as well as some gynecologic cancers.

Most often, radiation is not intended to cure cancer but rather make it more treatable through other means, either by reducing it in size or decreasing the likelihood that it will recur. Radiation may reduce the growth of cancer or lessen its symptoms, but it does not necessarily eliminate the disease completely.

Chemotherapy

A more recent development than surgery and radiation, chemotherapy—the use of drugs to destroy cancer cells—is also one of the mainstays of conventional cancer treatment. The discovery of chemotherapy was an indirect result of chemical warfare during World War I. Soldiers who had been exposed to mustard gas, a poisonous chemical used as a weapon, were later discovered to have low blood counts. Subsequent studies throughout the 1940s found that nitrogen mustard, a chemical compound in mustard gas, worked effectively against lymphoma, a cancer of the white blood cells centered in the lymph nodes. Nitrogen mustard served as the model for a series of chemical treatments (chemotherapy agents) that were developed to kill cancer cells by damaging their DNA. By the 1950s, the use of these cytotoxic agents was widely accepted and employed by the medical community as a standard treatment for various types of cancer. Then, in the 1960s, a new method of using chemotherapy called *combination chemotherapy* emerged. Doctors began to combine chemotherapy drugs to attack cancer cells at different stages of growth, thereby inhibiting the ability of the cells to overcome treatment. Combination chemotherapy continues to be used today.

According to the American Cancer Society, there are now nearly 100 chemotherapy drugs on the market. Although their uses differ, the drugs are similar in that they damage and kill the cancer cells they are designed to target. Unlike surgery and radiation, which are focal treatments and more commonly used for cancers that are localized, chemotherapy is usually administered systemically, meaning that it flows through your entire body, or system, killing cancer cells wherever they may exist. Although this seems simple and benign in theory, the practice of chemotherapy is problematic because, like radiation, the treatment may damage healthy cells, causing serious and even fatal side effects such as anemia, bleeding, and suppressed immunity, with consequent risk of infection, nausea, hair loss, and fatigue. These adverse side effects, in turn, make it necessary to limit the dosage of chemotherapy as well as the duration for which the treatment is used.

Chemotherapy is also imperfect in other ways. Frequently, cancer is able to build resistance to the treatment and eventually return. Even worse, some cancer cells (so-called cancer stem cells) are completely immune to the treatment. Therefore, in practice, chemotherapy does not lead to a cure for most cancers. Rather, it provides a temporary reprieve or period of stability for the patient.

Hormone Therapy

Although hormone therapy is not employed as frequently as surgery, radiation, and chemotherapy, it should still be considered a classical cancer treatment because of its use in the past. Theories about the connection between hormones and cancer emerged at the turn of the century—around the same time surgical techniques improved. In 1896, the British physician Sir George Beatson hypothesized that the female breasts were "held in control" by the ovaries, which led him to believe that the ovaries played a role in breast cancer development. Therefore, he surgically removed the ovaries of his female breast cancer patients.

Beatson's theory sparked interest in the medical community and was later expanded in the 1940s by Dr. Charles B. Huggins of the University of Chicago. Dr. Huggins put forward the theory that prostate cancer was connected to male hormone dysfunction and pioneered *male hormone (androgen) ablation,* a form of therapy designed to block

Specialized Cancer Therapies

The following cancer treatments fall into one of the categories of conventional therapy discussed in this chapter. Many are cutting-edge treatments that use tailored biology and advanced medical technology to destroy cancer cells and eliminate the disease from the body.

- **Cryosurgery.** Also called *cryoablation* and *cryosurgical ablation,* this is a minimally invasive cryotherapy (treatment involving cold temperatures) that destroys abnormal cells by freezing the tissue with liquid nitrogen, carbon dioxide, or argon gas.

- **Hyperthermia therapy.** A type of treatment in which body tissue is exposed to high temperatures to damage and kill cancer cells, or to make cancer cells more sensitive to the effects of radiation and certain anti-cancer drugs.

- **Intensity-modulated radiation therapy (IMRT).** A type of conformal radiation therapy that uses computer-generated images to outline a tumor's shape and size. By changing the intensity of radiation during treatment, the damage to surrounding healthy tissue is reduced.

- **Laparoscopic surgery.** This surgery, also known as laparoscopic-assisted resection, is performed with a *laparoscope*—a thin tube-like instrument with a light and lens for viewing. It may also have a tool to remove tissue to be checked under a microscope for signs of disease. This technique is frequently used in the treatment of gynecologic cancers.

- **Laser surgery.** A surgical procedure that uses the cutting power of a laser beam to make bloodless cuts in tissue or to remove tumors. This surgery is most often used to treat skin cancer but, on occasion, it has been employed for ovarian as well as head and neck cancers.

- **Microscopically controlled surgery.** This is a technique for removing certain cancerous tumors based on careful and precise microscopic control of the *surgical margins,* or the border of tissue surrounding the tumor. Originally conceived and implemented by Frederic Mohs, this procedure is also called *Mohs surgery* and *chemosurgery.*

- **Microsphere therapy.** This type of treatment involves the injection of *microspheres*—tiny, hollow, round particles made from materials such as glass, ceramic, or plastic—into blood vessels that feed a tumor to cut off its blood supply. Microspheres can also be filled with a substance (for example, radiation) that may help kill more cancer cells. Specialized types of this therapy include SIR-Sphere and Thera-Sphere.

- **Multidimensional conformal radiotherapy.** A specialized radiation treatment in which radiologic imaging and computer technology is used to match the beams of radiation to the size and shape of the tumor. A similar technique is known as *three-dimensional conformal radiation therapy* (3DCRT).

- **Oncolytic virus therapy.** A type of targeted therapy using a special type of virus that infects and breaks down cancer cells, but not normal cells. This therapy may make it easier to kill tumor cells with chemotherapy and radiation therapy. It is also referred to as *oncolytic virotherapy, viral therapy,* and *virotherapy.*

- **Photodynamic therapy.** A treatment using drugs that become active when exposed to light. These activated drugs may kill cancer cells.

- **Proton beam therapy.** A type of radiation therapy that uses streams of protons that are emitted from a special machine. This type of radiation kills tumor cells but does not damage nearby tissues. It is used to treat cancers in the head and neck, as well as in organs such as the brain, eye, lung, spine, and prostate.

- **Radiofrequency ablation (RFA).** A procedure that uses radio waves to heat and destroy abnormal cells. This technique, which can be effective even for cancers deep within an organ, is being used increasingly for liver tumors, and may be applied to lung and bone cancers as well.

- **Radioimmunotherapy.** A type of systemic radiation therapy in which a radioactive substance is linked to an antibody that locates and kills tumor cells when injected into the body.

- **Robotic surgery.** A surgical procedure performed with the aid of a robotic system controlled by a computer.

- **Sonodynamic therapy.** An experimental treatment that uses ultrasound to boost the cytotoxic (cancer-cell killing) effects of special drugs known as sonosensitizers.

- **Stereotactic radiosurgery.** Also called *radiation surgery*, this is a type of external radiation therapy that uses special equipment to position the patient and precisely administer a single large dose of radiation to a tumor. It is used to treat brain tumors and is being studied in the treatment of other types of cancer.

- **Transarterial chemoembolization (TACE).** A two-step therapy used in the treatment of liver cancer. Chemotherapy drugs are directly administered to the tumor via the artery that supplies blood to the liver, effectively targeting the cancer while avoiding side effects associated with whole-body chemotherapy. Following this treatment, the blood supply to the tumor is embolized, or cut off.

the production of male hormones, as a cancer treatment. His work eventually won him a Nobel Prize in 1966.

Today, hormone therapy remains a mainstay of breast and prostate cancer management, as well as a treatment for rare gynecologic and endocrine cancers. Unfortunately, hormone therapy is not effective for the majority of cancers, since there are not many types with a hormonal component.

MODERN CANCER TREATMENTS

Recent breakthroughs in the scientific understanding of cancer have given rise to more sophisticated treatment and dramatically expanded our arsenal of weapons against the disease—though our ability to manage the majority of cancers has, perhaps, improved less dramatically. Until the late 1990s, nearly all drugs used in cancer treatment (with the exception of hormone therapy) were chemotherapy drugs that killed cells in the process of replicating their DNA and reproducing. In the late 1990s, however, different types of anti-cancer drugs, such as rituximab (Rituxin) for lymphoma and trastuzumab (Herceptin) for breast cancer, became approved by the Food and Drug Administation (FDA). This breakthrough ushered in a new class of modern cancer treatment based on a "targeted" approach. Today, the term *targeted therapy* (see the inset on page 24) is commonly used to describe some of the latest treatments designed to hit a specific cellular target, such as a critical signal in a molecular pathway. But the term itself is broadly defined, which is why it may be more practical to classify the latest treatment methods by their respective modes of action. The next section discusses some of the recent advances in modern cancer therapy, which are categorized according to the biological action they take against cancer.

Immunotherapy

Immunotherapy is a type of cancer treatment that involves harnessing the patient's immune system. This concept is not new; in fact, it predates chemotherapy. Early forms of immunotherapy emerged around the same time as radiation therapy in the late nineteenth century. Dr. William B. Coley, working out of New York Cancer Hospital (which would later become Memorial Sloan-Kettering Cancer Center) observed spontaneous improvement in some of his sarcoma patients, a change he attributed to their recent bacterial infections. Dr. Coley suspected that these incidental infections had triggered the patients' immune systems, which, in turn, fought the cancer in addition to the infection. To test his hypothesis, Coley created a vaccine of dead bacteria and then administered it to his patients in hopes of reducing their tumors or eliminating them altogether. The experiment was met with some success, but overall, the results were inconsistent, making the treatment difficult to implement.[1] Upon Coley's death in 1936, the use of immunotherapy faded away, and radiation and chemotherapy took center stage as the preferred methods of cancer treatment.

The next major development came in the 1950s, when Drs. Thomas Lewis and McFarlane Burnet proposed the *tumor immune surveillance theory*, which suggested that all human immune systems have specialized white blood cells that continuously survey and

What Is a Targeted Therapy?

Targeted therapy involves a group of anti-cancer drugs that attack the disease by aiming at a particular weak point found in the cancer cells. In general, targeted therapies block the growth and spread of cancer by interfering with specific target molecules involved in tumor growth and progression—much like how keys fit in certain keyholes to unlock a specific door or chamber. But there are different kinds of targeted therapy, and each disrupts the growth and spread of cancer in a specific way.

Some targeted therapies, for instance, inhibit specific growth factors involved in cancer cell proliferation. These drugs, also called *signal transduction inhibitors,* were heralded as a sign of a new era in cancer treatment when they made their debut in the late 1990s. One such drug is trastuzumab, or Herceptin, which became FDA-approved in 1998 and is designed to treat tumors that overproduce a protein known as "HER2," which occurs in about 20 percent of women with breast cancer. Combination treatments of Herceptin and chemotherapy have shown to cut the recurrence rate of early-stage breast cancer in half, as compared with chemotherapy treatment alone.

Other targeted therapies affect gene expression or induce *apoptosis* (death) in cancer cells. One example is tretinoin (Vesanoid), which activates retinoic acid receptors in genes and is approved to treat certain leukemias. Some types of targeted drugs such as bevacizumab (Avastin) hinder *angiogenesis,* a process involving the development of blood vessels that can promote tumor growth. Moreover,

destroy cancer cells that appear in the body. The theory prompted clinical trials focusing on the body's immune response to cancer. Although they found that immunotherapy was effective for localized bladder cancer, as well as some cases of melanoma and kidney cancer, the trials yielded few meaningful results. However, the 1970s proved to be a turning point in cancer research, changing how immunotherapy was received and used by the medical community. In this decade, further insight into how immune cells interact and work against can-there are targeted therapies that act by helping the immune system to destroy cancer cells or by delivering toxic molecules to cancer cells. More than thirty targeted therapies are currently being investigated in clinical trials, and others are undergoing development in the laboratory.

Although initially hailed as "smart bombs" and making it to the cover of *Time* magazine in 2001, targeted therapies nevertheless have serious limitations. A June 2010 article by *New York Times* writer Andrew Pollack, "Therapies for Cancer Bring Hope and Failure," summarizes the development of targeted therapy to date. In the report, Dr. J. Leonard Lichtenfeld of the American Cancer Society reflects that scientists and doctors have "gone through a very rapid period of high expectations, maturation and disappointments. . . . I think there was almost a naïveté that if we could find the target, we would have the cure." Problems that arise with targeted therapy include not only adverse side effects but also drug resistance, which may result from prolonged use of targeted drugs. This is not to mention the fact that cancers have many different mechanisms, pathways, and secondary pathways, and thus many potential targets. A drug may hit its target, but this single target may be too narrow and specific to do much more than temporarily hinder the cancer. Blocking or destroying only one aspect of a cancer's circuitry may not be good enough if a tumor has "backup" circuits. Since cancer treatments ultimately work best in combination, the future of targeted therapy is *multi-targeted therapy,* which can be achieved by combining either multiple targeted therapies or targeted therapy with classical treatments.

cer allowed doctors to understand how cancer cells can be recognized, rejected, and destroyed. As a result, immunotherapy was once again resurrected as a viable cancer treatment almost one hundred years after Dr. Coley's original observations.

In general, there are two kinds of immunotherapy, passive and active. *Passive immunotherapy* refers to treatments that influence the immune system via monoclonal (man-made) antibodies or immune cells, which are produced in a laboratory rather than naturally manufactured in the body. The antibodies act like guided missiles to attack the cancer, and the specialized, lab-produced immune cells work like mercenaries to destroy cancer cells in the body. In contrast, *active immunotherapy* involves the direct stimulation of a patient's immune system to reduce or eliminate the cancer without the transfusion of cells or injection of antibodies.

Today, immunotherapy has greatly expanded and uses many different agents. There are antibodies such as trastuzumab (Herceptin) for breast cancer, as well as rituximab (Rituxin), which is effective against some lymphomas and leukemias. Natural and pharmaceutical *adjuvants*—agents that act as treatment enhancers—and molecules called *cytokines* may also be given to patients to further bolster their immune system. Additionally, cancer patients may be transfused with specific immune cells, including natural killer (NK) cells, dendritic cells, and gamma-delta T cells. And finally, there are vaccines and vaccination strategies that may employ some or all of the aforementioned agents to strengthen a patient's immune system so that the body can more effectively defend itself against cancer.

Immunotherapy is now considered one of the most promising approaches to cancer treatment. Dr. Louis Weiner, who heads the Lombardi Cancer Center at Georgetown University, has commented on the "remarkable potential of immunotherapy to eradicate cancer." Dr. Weiner summarized the current state of cancer immunotherapy particularly well in a recent article published in *The New England Journal of Medicine*, saying, "In 1987, an editorial . . . asked whether the field of immunotherapy was at the beginning of the end or the end of the beginning. In retrospect, I would say it was at the 'beginning of the beginning.'"[2]

Anti-angiogenic Therapy

Angiogenesis, a term consisting of the Latin words for blood (angio) and birth (genesis), is a word used to describe the formation and growth of blood vessels. *Anti-angiogenesis* is a therapy intended to halt this process by attempting to cut off the blood supply that feeds cancer cells, thereby disabling the disease and preventing further growth of the cancer.

Anti-angiogenic therapy is truly a modern concept. It was only in 1971 that Dr. Judah Folkman of Children's Hospital in Massachusetts published a seminal paper in *The New England Journal of Medicine* proposing that all cancers are dependent on a regular blood supply without which tumors would wither and die. At first, this theory was largely disregarded by the scientific community. It was not until 1989 that anti-angiogenic treatment became a reality. That year, Dr. Folkman reported the successful treatment of an angiogenesis-dependent disease using *interferon*, a cellular signal that interferes with the division of cancer cells and blocks tumor growth.[3] However, the first anti-angiogenic drug was not introduced to the market until 2004, when the FDA approved bevacizumab, or Avastin. (See page 74.)

Today, there are more than 300 anti-angiogenic substances—both natural and synthetic—that have been identified by scientists. A number of these substances are currently undergoing phase III clinical trials, and eight have been officially approved by the FDA as anti-cancer agents with recognized anti-angiogenic properties for a host of cancers, including breast, brain, and colon cancer. (See the inset on page 28 for more about clinical trials.)

Apoptotic and Epigenetic Therapy

Apoptosis, the Greek word for suicide, is defined as "programmed cell death" in biology. Healthy cells undergo this process as a natural part of their life cycle; they grow, differentiate (mature), and finally reach the point of apoptosis and die. However, when cells mutate and become cancerous, they lose the ability to undergo apoptosis. Therefore, *apoptotic therapy,* which is also called differentiation therapy, is meant to induce cell death in order to restore proper cellular function.

Scientists have known about the phenomenon of apoptosis for several decades, but it was not until the 1980s that they established the relationship between apoptosis and cancer development. Researchers discovered that the abnormal Bcl-2 gene, which is found in some lymphomas, interferes with apoptosis. Since then, medical scientists have learned that an array of genes—p53, p16, p21, p27, E2F, FHIT, PTEN, and CASPASE—as well as a complex set of molecular and cellular pathways and signals all affect a cell's survival and its process

What Is a Clinical Trial?

One of the keys to developing new cancer therapies is the clinical trial. There are many kinds of clinical trials—including prevention trials, screening trials, diagnostic trials, and quality-of-life trials—but the type most commonly referred to is the human treatment trial, which is used to test potential cancer treatments. Protocolized, structured, and expensive, the treatment trials process generally consists of four distinct phases to assess drug safety and effective dosages, establish treatment efficacy, and determine whether or not a new treatment is superior to the existing standard. These four phases are described below.

- **Phase I trials:** In these trials, an experimental drug or treatment is tested on a small group of usually twenty to eighty people to determine its side effects and safety, as well as its pharmacology.

- **Phase II trials:** In these trials, an experimental drug or treatment is administered to a larger group of up to 300 patients to assess its dosing and efficacy.

- **Phase III trials:** These are larger, randomized, and controlled studies of large groups of more than 300 people aimed at evaluating how effective the drug or treatment is when compared with the current standard.

- **Phase IV trials:** These are post-marketing studies done after a drug or treatment is approved. Scientists gather information regarding the effectiveness of the treatment, side effects, and how it should be optimally used.

If you are interested in learning more about this topic, the website of the US National Institutes of Health (www.clinicaltrials.gov) provides information in a question-and-answer format that is helpful and easy to understand. In addition, the National Cancer Institute's website (www.cancer.gov/clinicaltrials) is a valuable resource for information on trials specific to certain cancers.

of maturation and death. (See Figure 2.1 below.) Therefore, these genes may serve as potential targets for cancer treatment.

In order to repair malfunctioning genes and, therefore, restore a cell's innate ability to die naturally, a treatment known as *epigenetic therapy* was developed. "Epigenetic" means that the therapy focuses on gene function rather than simply gene structure, which is why it's so innovative. For a long time, medical scientists believed that cancer was caused by gene mutations—structural changes within the genes themselves. Only very recently have scientists and doctors realized that changes in gene function and expression may also affect cancer development and growth. Epigenetic therapy refers to treatments aiming to normalize genetic function. The first epigenetic drug for cancer, decitabine (Vidaza), was approved by the FDA in 2004. Remarkably, some of the leukemic patients who were given this drug saw a complete remission of their cancer.[4]

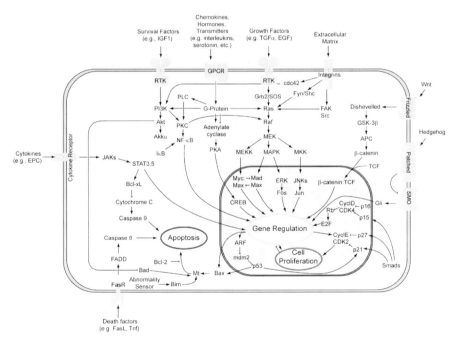

FIGURE 2.1. GENETIC SIGNAL TRANSDUCTION. An illustration of complex pathways involving specific genes like p53 and p21, as well as key protein molecules such as *capsases,* which play a role in the regulation of cell growth (proliferation) and death (apoptosis).

Other Therapies

In addition to immunotherapy, anti-angiogenic therapy, and apoptotic and epigenetic therapy, there are other interesting new treatments, targeting other biological and molecular pathways (such as the cellular process of *autophagy*), that are currently being researched. There are also therapies that take distinctive approaches, including cryotherapy, hyperthermia therapy, photodynamic therapy, and sonodynamic therapy, which target cancer cells using extremes in temperature, light, and sound, respectively. Other therapeutic approaches—including the use of oncolytic viruses to attack cancer cells and non-epigenetic gene therapies—are also in development. In time, other approaches to treating cancer will undoubtedly surface and add to an ever widening array of therapies against the disease.

CONCLUSION

The conventional treatments discussed in this chapter, both classical and modern, are all important weapons in the fight against cancer. Unfortunately, they are not as effective as medical scientists had hoped. While adequate weaponry is undoubtedly important, *how* this weaponry is used is equally, if not more, significant. For the most part, the conventional treatment strategy for cancer involves using one or two classical treatments—surgery, radiation, chemotherapy, or hormone therapy—one after the other. Only on occasion are different treatments used in combination simultaneously, such as when radiation and chemotherapy are administered following a patient's surgery to prevent the recurrence of cancerous tissue. Moreover, modern treatments like immunotherapy (as well as others discussed in this chapter) are employed only when classical treatments are ineffective.

Although there are other strategic options, the dominant approach to cancer treatment continues to be mostly one-dimensional. Later in this book, I will propose a new multi-treatment "cocktail" method, which may hold the key to successful cancer therapy. But first, we need to examine the theory behind the current approach to treating cancer and understand why it is insufficient.

3

Conventional and Cocktail Strategies for Cancer Treatment

We are not lacking in cancer therapies. As outlined in the previous chapter, there are now novel treatment methods such as immunotherapy, anti-angiogenic therapy, and apoptotic and epigenetic therapy in addition to the classical treatments—surgery, radiation, chemotherapy, and hormone therapy. Although these "weapons" may assist us in fighting the war on cancer, they do not necessarily guarantee a victory. Could it be that we are losing the war on cancer not because of inferior weaponry, but because of an inadequate and misguided strategy? This chapter offers a possible answer to this question, first by examining the theory behind existing treatments, and then by introducing a promising alternative—cocktail therapy. A closer look at the rationales behind these opposing strategies will further highlight the need to think beyond the magic bullet.

REDUCTIONISM IN WESTERN BIOLOGY AND MEDICINE

The current treatment strategy for cancer is based on the early, simplistic understanding of the disease as unabated cell growth, and is modeled after the successful treatment of infectious diseases. Modern science and medicine is guided largely by *reductionism,* a philosophy based on the idea of trimming a complex "whole" down to its simpler individual parts in order to understand it. This mode of thinking is entrenched in classical scientific thought in the Western world and dates back to ancient Greek philosophy. Democritus (460–370 BC), who is widely considered the father of modern science, proposed the idea that all physical changes in the world are caused by changes in the motion of microscopic atoms, which came to be known as the atomic theory. According to this theory, nature is a complex machine consisting of smaller entities working together. Following this philosophical tradition, the famous seventeenth-century philosopher René Descartes argued that the world was like a machine with a clockwork mechanism that could be understood by examining its smaller parts. This theory also extended to animals, including humans. Figure 3.1 (see below), which depicts a mechanical duck, reflects Descartes' philosophy that the bodies of animals are nothing more than complex machines, and that bones, muscles, and organs can be likened to cogs, pistons, and cams. This reductionist way of thinking still serves as the basis for many areas of modern science, including biology and medicine.

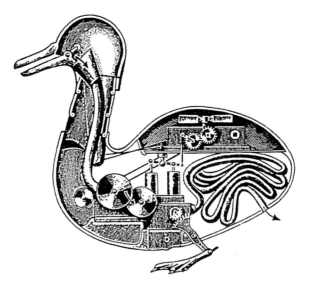

FIGURE 3.1. VAUCANSON'S FAMOUS DUCK. A mechanical duck designed by the French engineer Jacques de Vaucanson in 1737. The invention was intended to both demonstrate and perform the process of digestion. Although digestion did not take place, this famous duck reflects the reductionist principle that animals can be thought of as machines.

Since modern biomedical understanding has been shaped by reductionism, current treatment strategies for many diseases are also heavily influenced by it. Reductionist medicine is based on the simplistic notion that a disease can be cured or controlled by identifying the cause of the disease, and then finding treatments to eliminate the determined cause. The fact that this strategy works for many conditions, including diabetes, hypertension, and common infections, has tended to affirm its universality as a strategic principle—at least until the advent of HIV, which demonstrated that simple single-agent treatments are inadequate for controlling complex diseases. (See page 39 to learn about HIV treatment.)

Historically, cancer therapy adopted its principal treatment strategy from the successful reductionist model for infectious disease—a single cause is identified, a single treatment is looked for, and a single treatment results in a cure. For example, in 1930, conjunctivitis in infants was cured with penicillin, which killed the susceptible *Neisseria gonorrhea* bacteria that caused the infection. The same principle was applied to the initial treatment of syphilis, malaria, and tuberculosis using penicillin, quinine, and streptomycin, respectively. This success reinforced the viability of this approach: Identify the cause of the disease, and then use the right treatment to cure it.

The logic underlying conventional cancer therapy developed along a similar course, as scientists attempted to identify the cause of cancer and develop treatments that specifically targeted the cause. The rationale was as follows: If excessive cell growth was the cause of the disease, effective treatment would simply stop the cell growth. This is the essential logic behind chemotherapy, just like antibiotics for infections. Indeed, the parallel between infectious disease and cancer treatment is not incidental; even the term "chemotherapy," as coined by Paul Ehrlich (1854–1915), originally described the use of chemicals to kill germs. It is also worth noting that Ehrlich—a Nobel Prize winner credited with curing syphilis and founding modern immunology and chemotherapy—is the same brilliant scientist who popularized the concept of "magic bullet" cures for diseases. (See the inset on page 34.)

However, applying reductionist principles to cancer leaves us with simplistic definitions of the disease as well as simplified strate-

The Origins of the "Magic Bullet" Cure

Originally inspired by the German folktale of Der Freischütz ("The Devil's Bullet"), the renowned scientist and Nobel Laureate Paul Ehrlich outlined the "magic bullet" theory in a lecture presented to the Royal Institute of Public Health in London in 1907. In the lecture, he described the potential of drugs to pinpoint a bacterium or virus, destroy it, and leave all healthy cells untouched—hence, a "magic bullet." Since then, the term has been widely adopted to imply treatments and drugs that can deliver a seemingly magical cure.

gies for treatment. For a long time, cancer was simply defined and understood as the unchecked growth of cells, mutated genes, or signaling errors in cellular pathways. This calls to mind the ancient tale of the blind men and the elephant, in which a group of blind men attempt to identify an elephant based on the part of the animal they touch. The man who touches the tail identifies the elephant as a rope; the man who touches the ear says it is a fan; and the men who touch the leg and wall guess that the elephant is a pillar and a wall, respectively. This story reflects the limits of reductionism: Individual parts do not necessarily provide or allow knowledge of the whole. Also, we now know that cancer is a diverse, complex, and dynamic condition involving multiple pathways and many levels of biological function—it cannot be simply defined. As such, perhaps our current therapy strategies, which are based on former reductionist and overly simplistic understandings of cancer, should be revamped.

REDUCTIONISM, MONOTHERAPY, AND CANCER TREATMENT

The current strategy for treating cancer has been influenced by reductionist principles and, therefore, is based on the treatment model for infectious diseases like syphilis and strep throat. Conventional cancer treatment is generally straightforward and falls into the category of *monotherapy*, a term used to describe therapy in which treatments are administered one at a time in a linear fashion. The typical treatment strategy in monotherapy involves first reducing the disease volume as much as possible via surgery, radiation, or chemotherapy, perhaps with additional modalities, such as hormone therapy, to enhance the treatment's effectiveness. If this fails, or if the cancer progresses or recurs, further treatments may be given either one at a time or in a simple combination—depending on the type and nature of the cancer—to see if any one of them is effective.

A good example is the standard management of localized prostate cancer. Surgery or radiation is first applied to rid the prostate of cancer cells, which is then followed by a period of hormone therapy to suppress the cancer or prevent its recurrence. Thereafter, if the cancer returns, other hormone regimens or chemotherapy may be attempted. The same logic and strategy are followed for the treatment of many early-stage cancers, including breast and colon cancer.

To use an analogy, monotherapy can be likened to trying one key after another to open a lock. The approach is sequential: treatment A is used first, followed by treatment B, treatment C, and so on. The "magic bullet" logic is so overpowering that it dominates the strategy for modern cancer treatment, as indicated by a 2001 editorial in the prestigious *New England Journal of Medicine,* "A Magic Bullet for Cancer—How Near and How Far?" The editorial is aptly titled, reflecting the widespread fantasy of the medical community's quest for a magic bullet.

There are apparent practical advantages to the simplistic one-key/one-lock approach, in addition to its obvious success in the treatment of other diseases. First, applying one drug or regimen at a time allows doctors to chart statistics and see how well a particular treatment works. When several drugs are administered at once, it becomes difficult to pinpoint the one that is effective. Additionally, when one treatment is used at a time instead of multiple treatments, side effects are kept to a minimum. If a side effect does occur, doctors can identify the exact agent that caused it.

There are also many peripheral reasons contributing to the predominance of monotherapy. For instance, the modern medical system is highly protocolized, so the process of discovering, approving, and prescribing new drugs is tightly regulated and formalized. A less obvious but nevertheless powerful influence is the cost of cancer therapy, as well as the ensuing reluctance of insurance companies to subsidize treatments that are not standard or FDA-approved. And this is not to mention the fact that the simultaneous use of multiple treatments would dramatically increase the cost. Moreover, the medical establishment's bias against so-called alternative treatments also makes it less likely that they will be used in place of or alongside conventional treatments. Finally, concerns about liability make cancer doctors hesitant to prescribe out of the established routine, thereby limiting how many treatments will be used at any one time.

All practicalities aside, we should seek a better and more effective strategy for cancer treatment, since it is obvious that our current approach is not producing ideal results. Could it be that some of the assumptions underlying the one-key/one-lock approach to treatment are fundamentally flawed? It is possible that we have incorrectly assumed that there is only one "lock," which has led us to believe that opening the lock—curing cancer—is just a matter of finding the right key. Another possibly false assumption is that we have or eventually will have the right key. But what if there are multiple locks or combination locks instead? And what if there is no perfectly fitting, "right" key to be found? This would mean never opening the lock, no matter how many keys we try. Therefore, it is time to consider an entirely new strategic approach in which multiple keys are tried and used simultaneously in order to address a potentially "multi-lock" situation.

THE COCKTAIL STRATEGY FOR CANCER TREATMENT

Cancer biology is complex, as you already know. Monotherapy may be too simplistic a strategy to treat the disease effectively, which is why a complete rethinking of the conventional approach is needed. Based on what we know about the multifaceted, multi-pathway biology of cancer, a better strategy is one based on the dynamic and simultaneous use of diverse agents, including drugs, vitamins, herbs, and diet, in order to overwhelm the disease. The logic underlying this approach may yield better results, and there is a growing body of scientific research that supports this strategy. Moreover, a multifaceted, or "cocktailed," approach to treating disease is not without precedent in non-Western traditions and modern medicine alike. The next section looks at some of the models and rationales for the cocktail treatment strategy.

Traditional Chinese Medicine

It is important to understand that monotherapy is not universal, just as Western medicine is not the only way to effectively treat disease. Researchers and physicians trained in the Western tradition have reductionist ways of thinking instilled in them from the moment they begin their scientific education. Yet, this mode of thought is not necessarily a norm in other medical traditions, in which the use of multiple-ingredient therapies and complex compounds is common, and even routine.

In Asia, basic concepts of health and illness developed much differently than in the West. Illness was seen as an imbalance of complex forces in the body that manifested as symptoms.[1] Traditional Chinese Medicine (TCM) developed around this core principle. As a result, the mainstay treatments of TCM involve the dynamic use of herbal concoctions, or patent formulas ("Fu-Fang"). These formulas are a combination of substances such as herbs, minerals, and marine and land animal parts. Each ingredient contains biologically active compounds that may have different effects in the body. Herbal formulas are even used for simple conditions like the common cold or flu, and their contents may change over the course of treatment in order to respond appropriately to the diverse, variable nature of disease. The fundamental goals of TCM pharmacology are not only enhancing the efficacy of treatment via the strategic combination of ingredients, but also producing *synergy*—a phenomenon in which a combination of different elements produces greater effects than any one element alone. (See page 44 for more information about synergy.)

Another key characteristic of Traditional Chinese Medicine is its unique conception of the human body, which is visualized as having multiple "points" for treatment to target. As an example, the practice of acupuncture involves the insertion and manipulation of thin needles in any of an individual's 400 points along the body's energy channels, of which there are 20. (See Figure 3.2, below.) The combination of points stimulated produces a certain effect in the body in order to treat a particular condition. The multidimensional aspect of acupuncture makes it another example of cocktail therapy.

Modern Integrative Pain Management

There are also areas of modern Western medicine in which various medications may be combined to produce a better outcome than a single agent could achieve alone. This cocktail approach is prominent

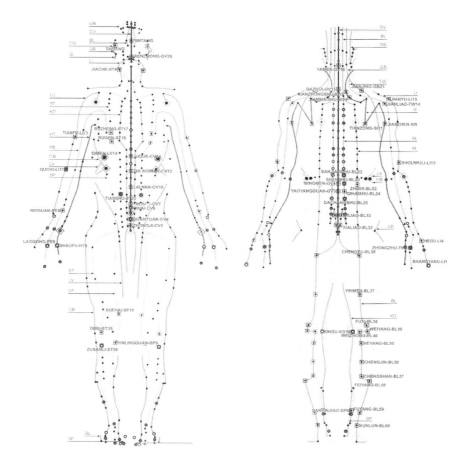

FIGURE 3.2. A MULTIDIMENSIONAL APPROACH TO TREATMENT. The multiplicity of energy points and channels in the body, as conceived by Traditional Chinese Medicine. In acupuncture therapy, these points are stimulated simultaneously, implying a cocktailed approach to treating disease.

in the field of pain management. Common analgesics (painkillers) such as narcotics and nonsteroidal anti-inflammatory drugs, also called NSAIDs, may be combined with atypical agents, including antiepileptic drugs, antidepressants, muscle relaxants, glutamate receptor antagonists, acupuncture, cold packs, heat therapy, massage, hypnosis, and even music to enhance overall pain relief.

In the related field of anesthesia, particularly general anesthesia, multiple agents are frequently required as well. These include hypnotic drugs or analgesics (midazolam or propofol), opioids (meperidine), paralytic drugs (vecuronium), and an inhaled general anesthetic such as halogenated ether (sevolurane and desflurane). Applied in a thoughtful, rational, and systematic manner, the combination of multiple agents has not only been used in Western medicine, but also proven to be a superior therapeutic approach.

Modern HIV Treatment

The best example of a successful combination approach in Western medicine is the case of HIV treatment, which evolved from monotherapy to cocktail therapy over the course of two decades. It was not that long ago when the human immunodeficiency virus (HIV) was universally believed to be fatal, and an AIDS diagnosis was comparable to a death sentence. In the United States alone, more than 60,000 people died of AIDS between 1981, when the condition was first described, and 1987, when treatment first became available. The average survival rate for AIDS in the 1980s was less than two years, despite improvements made in the management of the disease and the development of azidothymidine (AZT), an antiviral drug specifically targeting HIV.[2] In contrast, recent reports indicate that people diagnosed with HIV today can expect to live twenty-five years on average. So what happened? Did scientists find a magic bullet? Was it simply the discovery of new drugs? In actuality, it was a new treatment *strategy*—in addition to new drugs—that revolutionized HIV therapy, changing it from a deadly disease to a chronic one.

In line with the tradition of treating infectious disease with one antibiotic after another, standard treatment for HIV between 1987 and 1995 followed the one-drug-at-a-time approach. But it didn't take long for scientists like Dr. David Ho and his team to figure out that "numerology. . . predicted that we would have a great deal of difficulty treating the virus with a single drug, and . . . essentially predicted the doom of monotherapy." Here, Dr. Ho is referring to the ability of the virus to mutate and become resistant to treatment. Statistically speaking, the chances were high that a single-agent regimen would eventually fail due to the sheer number of viral mutations—there was bound to be one that could overcome or dodge any single drug. The only way around this problem was to use multiple drugs, thereby reducing the chance that a virus would mutate or evolve and become drug-resistant. An excerpt from a CNN interview with Dr. Martin Markowitz, an oncologist and Dr. Ho's collaborator, further clarifies this idea: "Think of the [virus] as being a jumper. And if you expose it to a hurdle, a low hurdle, one drug, it can jump over it eventually. . . . If you're going to treat this [infection] successfully, you really have to give it a lot of drugs simultaneously at the same time, upfront, really push for a cure. You don't wait and play with it. It'll kill the host. . . . Similarly, if you play with [HIV], you'll just basically run out of drugs."

By 1995, Dr. Ho's team had initiated several programs of using a number of drugs in combination, each with a different mechanism or target, to treat HIV. This "cocktail" therapy lowered the AIDS mortality rate six-fold in developing countries and revolutionized modern treatment of HIV. For his innovative efforts, Dr. Ho was named Man of the Year by *Time* in 1996.

The HIV cocktail therapy devised by Dr. Ho has significant implications for cancer treatment, as there are many parallels between HIV and cancer. Both are incurable and deadly if left untreated. Both diseases are progressive and cause much physical misery for patients. Both involve mutations that can allow the virus and the cancer to escape treatment efforts. Although more so the case with cancer, both are complex diseases consisting of multiple targets for treatment. And while there is a wide array of drugs available for HIV and cancer, both conditions can be very expensive to treat.

Yet, there is a huge difference in the diseases' respective treatment success rates: Whereas people with AIDS today can look forward to many quality decades, most cancer patients do not survive. This difference in outcome is due not only to the difference in available therapies, but also the difference in treatment strategy. While cocktail therapy is now the standard treatment for HIV, monotherapy has, by and large, remained the status quo for cancer patients.

CONCLUSION

Just as there are different models for understanding the nature of our universe, from Newton's physics to Einstein's relativity, there are different models of medical treatment that vary by disease as well as culture. As demonstrated by monotherapy and cocktail therapy, how the biology of disease is understood significantly shapes the treatment strategy. Although it has yet to be used widely in Western medicine, cocktail therapy is a major component of non-Western medical traditions such as Traditional Chinese Medicine, and it has been employed in some areas of modern medicine as well. Multimodal pain management strategies illustrate how the cocktail approach can be viable and effective, and current HIV therapy serves as a poignant example of how the strategy has revolutionized treatment of a once-deadly disease. From these examples, we have learned that, sometimes, it is not a matter of finding magic bullets or better drugs, but rather using what already have in a better way—finding a magic strategy. In the next chapter, we will explore the cocktail approach to cancer treatment in more detail, beginning with its scientific rationale.

4

The Pros and Cons
of the Cocktail Strategy

There are simple medical conditions such as strep throat and acne, and there are complex diseases such as AIDS and cancer. Straightforward tactics and solutions may suffice for simple conditions, but this is not the case for complex conditions like cancer, which affects multiple body sites, arises at different stages, and produces diverse symptoms and other physical disruptions. Cancer has multiple biological targets for which no magic bullets are known, and for which the effectiveness of any particular treatment remains limited. This situation may call for a dynamic cocktail strategy in order to achieve superior outcomes. The first half of this chapter looks at the reasons why superior results can be achieved with a combination approach. Then, the second half focuses on some of the concerns currently preventing this strategy from being implemented and, therefore, paving the way for a potential cancer cure. As you will find out, by applying cocktail therapy in a pragmatic way, the obstacles we are facing can be overcome.

THE PROS OF COCKTAIL THERAPY

We have already seen that conventional medical practice has successfully treated simpler diseases, such as infections that require a single antibiotic. In general, the same straightforward treatment strategy has been applied to cancer therapy. But there are distinct advantages to using an alternative approach—the cocktail strategy. Some of these advantages are highlighted below.

Additive Advantage

In any situation, additive advantage can be simply defined as, "one plus one equals two." To illustrate, if a student's chance of being accepted to one college is approximately 15 percent, it makes sense to apply to multiple schools at once in order to increase the likelihood of acceptance. It would not make sense to apply to only one school, as the student then risks being rejected and having to wait a full term to apply again. Similarly, cancer therapy can be approached by simultaneously applying multiple treatments, each with a certain rate of effectiveness, to achieve a greater chance of success. To put it more simply, if treatments A, B, and C each have a 15-percent chance of being successful, then they have a 45-percent chance of success when used together, assuming the treatments do not cancel each other out. In this example, a combination approach *triples* the likelihood of treatment effectiveness.

Furthermore, though the chance of acceptance to a particular school may be average, the likelihood of acceptance increases when a student applies to many schools simultaneously. Of course, this strategy may not be necessary if the student (or, in the case of cancer, the patient) has a 90-percent chance of acceptance (treatment success). It is also not necessary to use this approach if time is not a factor, such as in the event that a student does not mind re-applying to colleges term after term, or if a relatively short delay in treatment (due to chronic conditions such as high cholesterol, for example) does not have any serious consequences. Unfortunately, current treatments for cancer are, generally speaking, not very effective, so delays in treatment could be a matter of life and death.

Synergy

The ancient Greek word *synergos* referred to multiple parts working together, and today we use the term *synergy* to imply different entities or energies cooperating to produce an optimal or better outcome.

Synergy occurs when a combination of individual parts works to enhance the effectiveness of each other, resulting in greater benefits. This idea can also be stated as, "one plus one is *greater than* two." For example, social synergy takes place when people with different skills work together to achieve a better community than individual contributions are able to achieve. Synergy is also a common concept in pharmacology, as drugs interact in ways that can enhance or magnify therapeutic effects. An everyday example is when aspirin or acetaminophen works in synergy with codeine to provide better pain relief, which is why drug combinations are sometimes prescribed for pain management. Thus, treatments A and B working together synergistically are more effective than either A or B used alone, as well as A and B used additively. So, theoretically, multiple drugs and treatments can produce multiple synergies, thereby making the overall therapy much more likely to succeed. For example, patent formulas in Traditional Chinese Medicine are based on the concept of creating synergies among the individual herbal ingredients.[1] There is also abundant scientific evidence that synergies can be produced among anti-cancer drugs and other treatments.

Synergy is produced in cancer therapy when chemotherapy enhances radiation to elicit a better response in the patient, as chemotherapy agents can sensitize the cancer cells to radiation. Synergy can also be produced among various chemotherapy agents that take action against different aspects of the cell growth cycle. There are synergies between chemotherapy and immunotherapy, as well as radiation and immunotherapy, since low-dose chemo and prior radiation can make immunotherapy more effective. There are even potential and demonstrable synergies between conventional and alternative treatments, which will be explored in more detail in Chapter 6. (See page 76 for a list of synergistic treatments that include unconventional therapies.) For now, here are some examples of potential synergies within and between conventional treatment modalities:

- Chemotherapy + radiation[2]
- Anti-angiogenic therapy + chemotherapy *or* immunotherapy or radiation[3]
- Chemotherapy + immunotherapy[4]

- Radiation and immunotherapy[5]
- Radiation + immunotherapy + anti-angiogenic therapy[6]
- Radiation + epigenetic therapy[7]

Tipping Point Potential

A *tipping point* is the critical turning point in a situation causing a radical turn of events. The term is also used to describe a very small change that has dramatic consequences. This idea is similar to the domino and avalanche effects and is a relatively new word in our language, coined in 1957 by a social scientist. "Tipping point" now refers to almost any change that is likely to have extraordinary effects. The implication is simply that seemingly small forces can cause a situation to tip over in a big way because a critical point has been reached. To illustrate, imagine a feather landing on one end of a finely balanced scale and causing it to tip, or a small boy joining a tied match of tug-of-war and influencing the outcome of the game. Or, to return to the college application analogy, it may not be the grades, test scores, and recommendation letters that "tip the scales" in favor of admission, but rather the warm, confident smile during the interview. In medicine, the tipping point can occur in a situation in which a combination of treatments goes beyond additive and synergistic effects to produce a critical response.

In terms of cancer treatment, the tipping point concept can be applied to a situation in which seemingly insignificant or inconspicuous interventions—such as the addition of a vitamin or special diet—causes the cancer to regress. The medical literature contains numerous reports of so-called "spontaneous" regressions of cancer in which there is a reversal of the disease even though treatment to bring about this change has not knowingly been used.[8] This phenomenon may be attributed to the tipping point effect. Like acceptance to college, cancer survival is an either/or situation; the cancer either recurs or it does not, and a patient either survives or does not survive. Theoretically, even a minor intervention or treatment can tip the scales and determine the outcome. Seemingly insignificant treatments—such as vitamins, diets, and even changes in mental attitude—can not only make *a* difference, but also sometimes *the* difference.

To state it another way, a combination of therapies may achieve the critical mass needed to subvert the disease and reverse the tide. And since we do not know what particular intervention will tip the scales in any one cancer case—just as we do not know what factor in a student's college application will secure admission—it logically follows that a combination of potentially effective therapies may increase the chances that a tipping point is reached.

Time Saving

When it comes to cancer, sometimes timing is everything. Frequently, a patient cannot afford to wait and see if a certain treatment will work, since the disease's natural course is to progress—or at least put the patient at risk for a certain period of time. Very often, by the time doctors learn that a certain treatment is not working, the patient has already lost a valuable treatment window. In other words, the cancer may have progressed to such a point that applying another treatment becomes difficult, if not impossible. It is obvious that if a particular treatment takes six weeks to prove beneficial or not, trying two treatments may take twelve weeks. But if the treatments are used simultaneously, the time required is cut in half. Therefore, another reason to apply treatments at once and right away is to minimize the time that is needed to determine their effectiveness and achieve a positive response.

Reduced Resistance to Treatment

In many cases, conventional cancer treatment can initially beat back the disease. However, as the same treatment is applied again and again, cancer cells may adapt to the treatment and, over time, develop resistance against it. This is why chemotherapy fails in many instances. Similarly, viruses like HIV tend to build resistance to antibiotics over time in a phenomenon known as *drug resistance*. You may recall that Dr. David Ho identified this problem as the main reason for deploying cocktail therapy against HIV. Simultaneously applying multiple treatments, especially when they are from different drug classes and act via different biological mechanisms, can dramatically reduce the likelihood that a virus or cancer will develop resistance. This, in turn, leads to improved patient responses and treatment efficacy, and increases the likelihood that the cancer will be cured.

An example of this is *multidrug resistance* (MDR), which was discussed in Chapter 1 (see page 11). When the MDR-1 gene is overexpressed in a cancer cell, it overproduces the substance P-gp, which pumps anti-cancer treatments out of the cell. To get around this problem, doctors can combine cancer treatments with substances that can overcome or reverse MDR or target P-gp.[9] Although new drugs are being developed and investigated for this purpose, existing drugs and herbs may also have the ability to overcome drug resistance and, therefore, could be combined with conventional therapies to improve treatment outcomes.[10]

Improved Quality of Life

Besides its potential to enhance treatment effectiveness, a combination approach may also reduce side effects and improve patients' quality of life. Not only have various drugs been found and developed to reduce side effects from radiation and chemotherapy, but many non-drugs—including herbs, supplements, Traditional Chinese Medicine, homeopathics, acupuncture, aromatherapy, and mind-body techniques—have also been shown to help patients undergoing cancer treatment. These agents can reduce the toxicity of conventional treatment and improve overall quality of life.

It is obvious that there are many compelling and logical reasons to use a combination of therapies, which can work together to make treatment more effective. As it turns out, there are still some issues preventing doctors from adopting the cocktail approach. In order to move towards a more effective treatment strategy, these stumbling blocks should be examined.

THE CONS OF COCKTAIL THERAPY

As just discussed, there are many reasons why deploying multiple treatments in combination may enable better outcomes. But if the logic behind the cocktail strategy is so obvious, why is it not the standard for cancer treatment? This section takes a look at some of the objections to cancer cocktail therapy, explains why these objections are misplaced, and describes how they can be intelligently and rationally overcome.

Side Effects

The possibility of adverse side effects is perhaps the foremost concern among doctors. Oncologists are usually hesitant to combine more than one drug, since the risk for side effects increases along with the number of side effects that may occur. Furthermore, two of the main cancer treatments—chemotherapy and radiation—are already quite toxic, so how can doctors safely create a cocktail of so many toxic treatments together? After all, there is a limit on the number of chemotherapy drugs that can be administered at once, and treatments that have similar side effects (for example, chemo and radiation) should be limited as well, especially if they are being used at the same time. A patient's body may not be capable of sustaining additive toxicities. However, it is only the classical treatments of chemotherapy and radiation that produce such intensive side effects; not all cancer treatments share their high level of toxicity. If doctors use only therapies with toxicity profiles that do not overlap or add up, or better yet, treatments with minimal toxicity, side effects will not be a major concern. For example, adding immunotherapy to anti-angiogenic therapy, or adding a drug to a vitamin or acupuncture, is not likely to cause serious side effects.

Negative Interactions

Negative interactions between different treatments are frequently cited as the reason why patients should not take additional treatments, especially without the supervision of a healthcare professional. Adverse interactions between cancer treatments are a legitimate concern. For select oral chemotherapy drugs alone, a recent review found a total of 184 potential interactions, 40 of which were considered to have a potential negative impact on patients.[11] Chemotherapy patients should also avoid using aspirin and NSAIDs, as these drugs can further increase the risk of bleeding, which is already heightened by chemotherapy. Additionally, antioxidant vitamins (for example, A, C, and E) may reduce the effectiveness of chemotherapy and radiation, which is why many cancer centers advise patients against taking any vitamin or supplement while they are undergoing these treatments. However, it's important to note that not all vitamins are antioxidants; some, including vitamin D_3 (see page 133), even positively interact with radiation and chemotherapy.[12] Still, negative interactions between different treatments is a legitimate issue and one that has been controversial in the medical literature.[13,14]

The advice here is to stay clear of controversy and be guided by medical science, but not to abandon treatment combinations altogether. If there are scientifically valid concerns that one treatment may negate another, it is best to avoid it. The same logic should be followed when planning an anti-cancer cocktail for a patient: Doctors should use only those treatment agents that do not have potential negative interactions. This is something physicians and pharmacists look out for on a daily basis, since patients may be prescribed many drugs together if they have multiple medical conditions or a complex medical situation. Concerns about potential negative interactions should be guided by research and the medical literature, and solved by intelligent prescribing. It should not serve as a deterrent against cocktail therapy.

Treatment Burden

Treatment burden is essentially an issue of convenience. It is simply inconvenient for patients to take so many treatments simultaneously, in turn making it difficult for them to comply with their treatment regimen. Even so, the use of several treatments or drugs at once is very common. It is not at all difficult to imagine an older patient with cardiovascular risk factors, osteoporosis, and depression simultaneously taking antidepressants, a beta blocker, a calcium-channel blocker, a bone-saving bisphosphonate, a stomach-saving H2 blocker, baby aspirin, a multivitamin, a calcium-magnesium supplement, and laxatives. Perhaps the patient had a recent fall and, therefore, requires daily rehabilitation and regular appointments with an acupuncturist, or even a psychiatrist to help with his or her depression. A significant amount of time is spent dealing with medical treatment, but is it worth it? Is it necessary?

Treatment convenience is a practical matter, and the related issue of medical compliance is frequently in the hands of the patient. There is an inverse relationship between convenience and compliance: The more inconvenient a treatment regimen is, the less likely patients are to comply with it. Unfortunately, modern medicine is not entirely convenient because of the complexity, specialization, and technology involved. Take, for example, a cancer patient who is already nauseated from chemotherapy and is then given additional medications and supplements. Whether or not this patient can tolerate more pills is a real and practical concern, as well as whether or not the patient will have the energy to seek other forms of treatment, such as acupuncture and group therapy.

Although legitimate concerns, convenience and compliance must be considered within the context of the huge problem we are tackling. Yes, cocktail therapy comes with the potential inconvenience of additional pills, treatments, and monitoring, but cancer is often a matter of life and death—so temporarily giving up convenience may be worthwhile and necessary to beat the disease. On the other hand, hospitals and cancer centers can try to ease the burden by providing some other therapies like acupuncture on-site, or allowing such therapies to be more easily scheduled.

Cost

Modern anti-cancer drugs are expensive, and several prescriptions may not be affordable for some patients. An example of this comes from a recent report stating that combining medicines for aggressive forms of breast cancer dramatically improves treatment outcomes. According to data presented at the 2010 CTRC-AACR San Antonio Breast Cancer Symposium, a combination of lapatinib, trastuzumab, and paclitaxel can improve tumor response rates up to 50 percent for HER2-positive breast cancers. This number stands in contrast to the individual effectiveness of each agent, which is 20 to 30 percent. The problem, however, is that each of these drugs costs at least (and usually more than) $5,000 per month, and insurance companies often balk at subsidizing multiple treatments at once. Typically, a second treatment is covered only after the first has failed. Still, not all cancer treatments are as costly, and technological advances, insurance coverage, and expiring patents may eventually bring down costs. The high cost of cancer care nevertheless remains, as Dr. Neil Spector of the Duke Cancer Institute says, a "real consideration."

Lack of Trials and Evidence

One of the major arguments made by the conventional and academic medical communities against cocktail therapy is the lack of clinical trials clearly demonstrating the benefits of each potential combination. The quest for magic bullets has fostered a culture in which scientists, the pharmaceutical industry, and regulatory agencies alike look for and test one drug or regimen at a time. The concern is that testing multiple treatments simultaneously may complicate the results and make it difficult to tell which treatment is producing a particular benefit or side effect. For example, if you give penicillin to a patient with a sore throat and he or she gets better, it is safe to assume that penicillin cured the sore throat. But what if you gave the patient penicillin, vitamin C, and Chinese herbs, and he or she got better? There is no dilemma for the patient, whose sore throat is now gone; but there is a *scientific* dilemma for the researcher, scientist, or doctor who cannot pinpoint the specific agent that relieved the sore throat. Was it the penicillin, the vitamin C, the Chinese herbs, or all three?

Whether or not there is a practical way to test and validate treatment cocktails is also a question. To conduct scientifically valid trials of combination treatments, scientists would first need to show that treatments A and B are each individually effective against a particular cancer, followed by trials to demonstrate that combining treatments A and B is more effective than using either one alone. Further trials would then be required to prove that combining treatments A, B, *and* C is better than both A and B individually, as well as A and B together. This process would need to be repeated for every cancer for which scientists wanted to prove the treatment's efficacy, with every trial taking years to complete. Moreover, since clinical trials are extremely costly—taking a single drug from bench to approval is as much as $860 million[15]—testing so many possible combinations would make the process of developing and approving drugs practically impossible.

So, here we have a problem. On the one hand, there is the cancer patient, who simply wants to get better and cares little about what particular drug or treatment works to that end. On the other, there is the researcher-scientist-doctor, who needs to know the specific agent that has a positive effect. Here's how this conflict can be resolved: Doctors and scientists should continue their scientific quest to understand cancer and discover new treatments, as well as conduct clinical trials to evaluate the benefits (if any) of these treatments. At the same time, a more pragmatic approach based on the guiding principles of medicine should be adopted. To deal with the near impossible task of proving the effectiveness of every combination treatment before implementing it, doctors should simply follow the Hippocratic Oath, and "do no harm." These three words should be the guiding philosophy for all doctors. If a particular combination treatment may benefit a patient without being harmful, then its use is warranted—even if full trial evidence is not yet available.

THE REALITY OF CANCER TREATMENT TODAY

At this point, a cancer patient may say, "But cancer therapy already uses combination treatments; my doctor says he will be giving me combination chemotherapy, and that's after receiving radiation and surgery to boot. So what's new about combination treatment for cancer?" Indeed, as early as the 1960s, chemotherapy evolved from single agents to combined and cyclically deployed regimens. Examples of combination chemotherapy include VAMP (vincristine, amethopterin, 6-mercaptopurine, and prednisone), which proved successful in the treatment of childhood leukemias.[16] More recently, the addition of non-chemo drugs such as rituximab (Rituxin) and bevacizumab (Avastin) to chemotherapy has shown to significantly enhance the treatment of some cancers.[17]

So, yes, combining drugs in cancer treatment is a growing trend. When I glance at a medical journal these days, a good percentage of the articles contain the word "combination." And it was not all that long ago, in June 2006, when *Time* magazine ran a feature entitled, "How Drug Cocktails Are Changing the Way We Treat Cancer." The article said that "doctors may have to become molecular chefs, cooking up new anti-cancer recipes with a growing number of promising drug ingredients." This is our vision, but treatment protocols and drug trials evolve very slowly in medicine. The day-to-day reality of current cancer treatment shows that cancer doctors are not yet the futuristic "molecular chefs" cooking up new recipes due in part to the following reasons:

- For the most part, modern cancer management does not involve *concurrent* treatments, but rather *sequential* treatments. In other words, most cancers today are still treated with one modality or treatment regimen at a time.

- Most of the combination regimens used today involve only approved pharmaceutical drugs. Some doctors may still have difficulty keeping an open mind about off-label drug usage, not to mention alternative treatments such as vitamins and herbs.

- Most new combination treatment regimens involve no more than two or three drugs, which frequently have similar mechanisms of action. Such is the case with combination chemotherapy. These combinations are simply nowhere near as expansive as the anti-cancer cocktail therapy envisioned and put forth in this book.

- Due to the high cost of cancer therapy, insurance companies nowadays are reluctant to cover the next line of treatment until the first regimen demonstrably fails. As such, a linear step-by-step, one-punch-at-a-time approach is quietly enforced. Moreover, there is practically no coverage at all for unconventional treatments or alternative medicine, which makes cocktail therapy even more financially burdensome for patients.

Regrettably, concerns about treatment side effects and negative interactions, along with a laborious clinical trials process, regulatory bureaucracy, and financial obstacles, constitute the reality of cancer care today. These factors are holding us back from potentially more effective treatment. The majority of cancer cases continue to be treated with one regimen at a time consisting of two or three drugs at most. This is not the cocktail strategy that may promise superior results. In the case studies on page 173, I describe actual cocktail therapy programs for cancer that include multiple agents and modalities, from drugs, vitamins, and supplements to herbs and mind-body techniques, in order to attack multiple aspects of the disease simultaneously. These examples of cocktail therapy can serve as guides, providing the blueprint for a superior treatment strategy.

CONCLUSION

A complex situation warrants a complex response, and a combination lock requires a combination of numbers applied at once in order to open it. Monotherapy, or simple regimens and single modalities applied sequentially until they fail, is not an optimal strategy. A complete rethinking of our approach to cancer treatment is needed. In the next chapter, I outline a rational and practical cocktail strategy that simultaneously employs multiple drugs from different categories and with different biological mechanisms. Non-drugs such as herbs, vitamins, supplements, and other so-called alternative treatments are also included. This advanced cocktail strategy has the potential to revolutionize cancer therapy.

5

Implementing Cocktail Therapy for Cancer

N ow that you are familiar with the theory and logic behind cocktail therapy, we need to turn our attention to the practical details of the approach. This chapter looks at the possible components, both conventional and unconventional, of anti-cancer cocktails. The conventional dimension of cocktail therapy involves a combination of standard treatments, while the unconventional dimension includes different classes of alternative treatments, such as off-label drugs, supplements, and specialized diets. This information will better enable you to work with your doctor in designing and implementing a cocktail treatment plan.

THE CONVENTIONAL DIMENSION OF COCKTAIL THERAPY

The conventional treatments reviewed in Chapter 2 are mainstays of a successful anti-cancer cocktail. These mainstream treatments, which are generally defined by their respective anti-cancer mechanisms, include surgery, radiation, chemotherapy, hormone therapy, immunotherapy, anti-angiogenic therapy, and apoptotic and epigenetic therapy. Such treatments are considered conventional because of their established use, validation by clinical trials, sanctioning by the FDA, and coverage by health insurance plans. They also abide by the so-called "standards of treatment" (see inset on page 58), as well as the consensus of both cancer specialists and the medical community in general.

What Are "Standards of Treatment"?

Standards of treatment is a legal term in tort law referring to the degree of prudence required under a duty of care. In medical practice, it refers to guidelines that specify appropriate treatment based on scientific evidence as well as the collaboration of medical professionals involved in the treatment of a particular condition.

As you now know, conventional treatments are normally administered one after the other rather than in combination. For example, a patient with breast cancer may undergo surgery to remove the diseased breast followed by chemotherapy, then radiation, and then hormone therapy to reduce the risk of recurrence. There are, however, various conventional therapies that have been shown to work together both additively and synergistically, and are currently being studied. Examples of synergistic combinations were provided in Chapter 4, but they are worth listing again here:

- Chemotherapy + radiation[1]

- Anti-angiogenic therapy + chemotherapy *or* immunotherapy *or* radiation[2]

- Chemotherapy + immunotherapy[3]

- Radiation + immunotherapy[4]

- Radiation + immunotherapy + anti-angiogenic therapy[5]

- Radiation + epigenetic therapy[6]

Combinations of conventional treatments are not limited to the ones listed above—there are countless others that have produced superior outcomes. One case in point is the treatment of multiple myeloma, an incurable form of blood cancer. There are currently ten different treatments for the disease, which vary based on the stage of the cancer as well as factors specific to the individual patient. Up until the early 1990s, multiple myeloma was treated mainly with combination chemotherapy and/or corticosteroids. But, since 2003, various combinations of four new drugs have doubled the survival of myeloma patients. Today, a symptomatic patient who is not a candidate for a stem cell transplant may instead receive MPT or MPV, which is a combination of melphalan (chemotherapy), prednisone (a corticosteroid), and thalidomide (an anti-angiogenic drug) or Velcade (targeted therapy). This combination has proven more effective than older therapies. Furthermore, the most recent trials of combined targeted therapy and anti-angiogenic therapy (without chemotherapy) produced a remarkable 100-percent response rate for myeloma, suggesting that this combination is superior.[7]

In response to the excitement surrounding these advances in treatment, Dr. David Avigan of Beth Israel Medical Center at Harvard University commented that "success in myeloma treatment will ultimately come by hitting the disease from multiple angles [and] through different pathways [and] different vulnerabilities."[8] According to Dr. Avigan, this may involve combining targeted therapies with a stem cell transplant, followed by vaccinations and immunotherapy. This vision for myeloma treatment could be expanded and applied to all cancers to produce results that are potentially just as promising. Still, an optimal cocktail approach to cancer is one that is truly multidimensional; namely, it should include alternative treatments. The alternative, or unconventional, dimension of cocktail therapy is discussed in the next section.

THE UNCONVENTIONAL DIMENSION OF COCKTAIL THERAPY

Despite its popularity among patients, many conventional doctors may still be suspicious or disregard the use of alternative treatments for cancer, mainly because of their concerns about possible negative interactions and the lack of scientific proof for its effectiveness. With this in mind, let us first clearly define unconventional treatment.

Also called *alternative medicine,* therapies such as herbs, vitamins, supplements, meditation, acupuncture, and diets are unconventional in the sense that they are generally not prescribed by mainstream cancer doctors, sanctioned by the FDA, or covered by health insurance plans. The word "alternative" can have a negative connotation because it implies that a treatment is untested, unscientific, and an *alternative* to mainstream medicine. Often, alternative health practitioners take the position that alternative and mainstream forms of treatment are not only different, but also incompatible, and they are opposed to using conventional therapies. This book, however, envisions a comprehensive cocktail approach that includes *all* potentially effective treatments—it does not promote alternative medicine to the exclusion of conventional therapy.

In terms of cancer treatment, unconventional treatment does not include the standard drugs routinely used and prescribed by oncologists. Rather, unconventional therapies fall into different regulatory categories such as off-label drugs and supplements, and some—like diets and spiritual activities—are non-medical and unregulated. Yet, just because a therapy is not officially considered a cancer treatment does not mean that it lacks scientific or clinical validity. In fact, many unconventional therapies have the same biological and anti-cancer mechanisms as conventional cancer drugs, working just like any cytotoxic (toxic to cells), immunomodulatory, anti-angiogenic, or epigenetic treatment described in Chapter 2. In the following pages, we will review the five key elements of unconventional cancer therapy: (1) Off-label drugs; (2) vitamins, herbs, and supplements; (3) diets; (4) mental and spiritual approaches; and (5) other alternative treatments that do not fall into any of the aforementioned categories.

1. Off-Label Drugs

Off-label drugs, a group that contains some of the potentially most useful treatments for cancer, are pharmaceuticals prescribed by physicians for conditions other than those for which they were originally approved by the FDA. A common practice often covered by insurance, using off-label medications can be thought of as the unconventional use of conventional drugs. For example, the antidepressant bupropion (Wellbutrin) may be used for weight loss; the antiepileptic drug gabapentin (Neurontin) has been prescribed for migraines; aspirin can be used to treat warts; and so on.

When it comes to cancer treatment, approved drugs for one type of cancer are frequently used for another type, but the use of non-cancer drugs to treat the disease is far from typical. This is not due to a lack of scientific evidence, but a lack of appreciation for the potential usefulness of such medicines. In addition, regulatory constraints, legal concerns, and established treatment protocols prevent the use of off-label drugs in cancer treatment. The fact of the matter is that there is a large inventory of common and relatively nontoxic drugs, ranging from aspirin to sertraline (Zoloft), that may effectively work against cancer. See page 85 of Part 2 for a list of off-label drugs that may act as anti-cancer agents.

2. Vitamins, Herbs, and Other Dietary Supplements

Although vitamins, herbs, and supplements refer to different groups of compounds in the United States, they all fall into a legislative category separate from foods and drugs. This distinction was established by the Dietary Supplement Health and Education Act (DSHEA) of 1994. The sections below describe each group.

Vitamins

Required for human nutrition, *vitamins* are organic compounds that, in most cases, must be obtained from dietary sources; with the exception of vitamin D_3, they are not manufactured by the body. It was actually vitamin deficiency that led to the discovery of vitamins, as insufficient vitamin intake can lead to disease. For example, Egyptians discovered that night blindness, which may be caused by insufficient vitamin-A intake, could be cured by eating liver—a food that is rich in the vitamin. Similarly, lemon and lime, which contain vitamin C, were found to prevent scurvy, and fish oil was discovered to be a cure for rickets because it contains vitamin D.

In general, the vitamins required by humans can be divided into two categories, fat-soluble and water-soluble. There are four fat-soluble vitamins (A, D, E, K) and nine water-soluble vitamins (the eight B vitamins plus vitamin C). Essential to cellular function in one way or another, almost all vitamins have some relevance to cancer. However, the vitamins identified as therapeutically useful are mainly the fat-soluble type—A, D, E, and K. As for the water-soluble vitamins, whereas vitamin C has long been suspected to fight cancer, B vitamins do not seem to have significant anti-cancer properties—some may actually promote cancer growth. The one exception to this rule is vitamin B_{17} (also known as laetrile), though it is not actually a vitamin. Turn to page 107 of Part 2 for a list of dietary supplements, including vitamins, that may be effective for cancer treatment and prevention.

Herbs

Herbs are plants that are ingested and used for flavoring or medicinal purposes rather than as food. Containing bioactive compounds that may help to combat disease and improve health, herbs have long served as the basis of Traditional Chinese Medicine, as well as Ayurveda and other indigenous health systems. The medicinal use of herbs in Western culture is rooted in the Hippocratic (Greek) elemental healing system and was heavily influenced by Islamic culture during the Middle Ages.

Modern pharmaceuticals have their origins in crude herbal medicines, and many drugs to this day are extracted from raw herbs and then purified to meet pharmaceutical standards. The word "drug" actually comes from the Dutch word "droog," which literally means "dried plant." Today, there are approximately 7,000 compounds in the pharmacopeia that are derived from plants,[9] including aspirin, which comes from the meadowsweet plant. The list of dietary supplements that begins on page 107 includes herbs that may be effective for cancer treatment and prevention.

Other Dietary Supplements

A *dietary supplement* is a substance taken orally that contains key ingredients intended to supplement the diet. Ingredients may include vitamins, herbs, minerals, or amino acids, or substances such as enzymes, organ tissues, glandulars, and botanic derivatives like soy isoflavones and green tea polyphenols. Dietary supplements, which also include extracts and concentrates, can be found in many forms, including tablet, capsule, softgel, gelcap, liquid, and powder.

Most supplements have limited and specific uses. For cancer, some may be useful for reducing the overall risk, while others have proven to aid in the treatment of specific cancers. Certain supplements may be taken to improve the chance of cancer survival or help diminish side effects from treatments like chemotherapy. A list of dietary supplements that may be effective for cancer treatment and prevention begins on page 107 of Part 2.

3. Diets

The relationship between nutrition and disease is a vast topic. Diet undoubtedly plays a huge role in human health, as evidenced by decades of research conducted by Professor T.C. Campbell and many others in the field of nutrition.[10] It also goes without saying that dietary factors have greatly contributed to the modern-day cancer epidemic. Some scientists estimate that 30 to 40 percent of cancers and 35 percent of cancer deaths can be linked to dietary factors.[11] It is common knowledge that some foods, such as fruits and vegetables, can prevent certain types of cancer, whereas foods like red meat and alcoholic beverages may increase the risk. It follows, therefore, that diet should be integral to cancer prevention and treatment.

A general dietary approach that has proven effective against cancer is caloric restriction, also referred to simply as a low-calorie diet. Caloric restriction was connected to extended lifespan as early as 1909, when Moreschi discovered that tumors did not grow as well in underfed mice as in freely fed mice.[12] Then, in the 1930s, Mary Crowell and Clive McCay of Cornell University found that animals who were fed a reduced-calorie diet while maintaining micronutrient levels could live twice as long as expected.[13] In the following decades, not much research was done in this area. Cancer doctors tended to tell patients that they could eat what they wanted, but by the 1980s, knowledge had advanced enough that scientists began to more deeply explore the connection between calories and cancer. Today, we know that calorie expenditure (i.e., exercise) reduces the risk of the disease, and that the biological mechanisms affected by calorie restriction enhance the repair of DNA and diminish the oxidative damage to DNA. Additionally, the restriction of calories has a positive effect on insulin metabolism and may influence gene expression, which may help to improve cancer outcome.[14] A landmark twenty-year study finally demonstrated in 2009 that caloric restriction decreases the incidence of cancer in monkeys.[15] The only evidence still missing is human trials to show that caloric restriction can prevent and/or treat cancer.

In addition to low-calorie diets, there are specific dietary regimens that have been touted as cancer treatments and, in some cases, cancer cures. These include macrobiotics, Gerson therapy, the Livingston-Wheeler regimen, the Kelley-Gonzalez regimen, metabolic typing, raw food diets, and wheatgrass therapy. Each has its own theory, which may overlap or even contradict those of other dietary regimens. Some of the programs are quite dogmatic and burdensome, dictating very specific foods to eat and avoid—despite the fact that such rigid guidelines may not be supported by science. Moreover, advocates of certain diets recommend their particular program to the exclusion of other cancer therapies, including conventional treatments, citing anecdotal evidence of cancer survivors who followed the diet. Yet, they fail to mention those who succumbed to the disease even though they kept to the dietary regimen. To illustrate this dietary approach to cancer treatment, let's take a look at two examples, macrobiotics and Gerson therapy.

Macrobiotics is a modified version of the traditional Japanese diet, which was made popular among cancer patients in the West thanks to the work of Michio Kushi, a Japanese immigrant and founder of the Kushi Institute. The diet is part of the overall macrobiotic lifestyle, which is based on the traditional Eastern view that sickness stems from humans' failure to harmonize with nature. According to the macrobiotic philosophy, cancer and other diseases are "symptom[s] of modern society"[16] attributable to the typical Western diet, which is heavy in meat, sugar, and artificial and processed ingredients. Although in line with current science, this idea came as a shock when it was initially proposed decades ago.

The standard macrobiotic diet consists of whole grains (40 to 60 percent), vegetables (25 to 30 percent), beans and seaweed (5 to 10 percent), and miso soup (5 percent). Supplementary amounts of fruit, fish and other types of seafood, condiments and seasonings, and some beverages are also allowed. On the other hand, foods and beverages such as red meat, eggs, dairy products, chocolate, hot spices, sugar, coffee, and alcohol are discouraged. Scientifically speaking, there is no doubt that consuming more whole grains and fresh vegetables, while avoiding foods like red meat, can reduce the risk of cancer. Still, it is not clear whether or not following a diet like macrobiotics is therapeutic for those who have already been diagnosed with the disease.

One of the shortcomings of macrobiotics is that it has not evolved along with the scientific understanding of cancer. For instance, it has not incorporated turmeric, a highly beneficial spice, or vitamin D. The diet also does not seem to recognize the potential hazards of *phytoestrogens*, which are contained in soy and may contribute to some female cancers. Finally, there have been few studies reporting improvements in the longevity of cancer patients who practiced the macrobiotic diet.[17] Currently, there are no clinical trials to validate macrobiotics as a viable cancer treatment.

Another well-known dietary regimen is the *Gerson diet,* also called Gerson therapy. This diet shares some basic tenets with macrobiotics, as it advocates an elemental diet of fresh organic fruits and vegetables. However, many of its guidelines, which include coffee enemas and ingestion of raw liver juice, are even more burdensome. The diet also prohibits some foods—for example, mushrooms—that are actually proven cancer fighters, while promoting the consumption of other foods that may support cancer growth, such as liver. Thus, basic principles of Gerson therapy may not be entirely valid from a scientific standpoint.

There are a number of other diets that are similarly flawed in that they are not completely based on current science or validated by clinical trials. Many reject other cancer therapies as well.[18] This is not to say that the diets totally lack merit. After all, some of their core principles, such as eating more fruits and vegetables, are healthy and protective against cancer. In general, though, cancer patients should not rigidly follow any diet, especially in place of other treatments. If a special diet is recommended by a healthcare professional, it should always be relevant to the cancer being treated, such as a low-fat diet for prostate cancer. A diet is appropriate when it is a component of an overall strategy and treatment plan that includes both conventional and unconventional therapies. Diets should not be used as standalone cancer treatments.

4. Mental and Spiritual Approaches

Although often overlooked, mental and spiritual health is an important aspect of cancer therapy. With cancer comes the possibility of death, causing mental suffering in addition to physical suffering. Surviving the disease depends not only on medical interventions, but also the patient's will to live and survive.

The relationship between mental attitude and physical survival has been the focus of study for several psychotherapists. Viktor Frankl, a celebrated psychotherapist and Auschwitz death camp survivor, famously wrote about the significance of hope in face of adversity.[19] Lawrence LeShan, a prominent therapist specializing in cancer patients, also eloquently described the importance of the mind and spirit in improving both well-being and chances of survival. One of his most illustrative cases is "Carol," a highly successful executive of a large corporation who was diagnosed with advanced malignant melanoma. At the time of diagnosis, Carol hated her corporate life, disliked the ruthless ambition of her colleagues, and unconsciously feared becoming like them. After being diagnosed and informed of her poor prognosis, she sought therapy from Dr. LeShan, who helped her recognize how this negative attitude was hurting her. LeShan refocused Carol on what she loved most in life, which prompted her to recall an experience she had working with injured handicapped people during her college years. To the shock of both her family and her friends, Carol quit her job, sold her apartment, and went back to school to become a special education teacher. She also ended her appointments with Dr. LeShan. When they met again ten years later, Carol told LeShan why she had stopped therapy: "I've been much too busy living my life to have any time for such nonsense as cancer, psychotherapy, or you!"[20]

Anecdotes aside, there are numerous clinical studies that support the link between mental and spiritual well-being and immunological health.[21] Recent studies have also confirmed that psychological intervention may actually reduce the risk of cancer recurrence as well as prolong cancer survival.[22] As such, a positive attitude and a will to overcome the disease form a vital cornerstone of cocktail therapy for cancer.

5. Other Alternative Treatments

There is a potpourri of unconventional cancer treatments that do not easily fall into any of the four previous categories. These include foreign treatments not readily available in the United States, such as lentinan (a Japanese mushroom derivative), mistletoe, and the Newcastle Disease Virus (NDV), as well as unapproved or outlawed drugs like dichloroacetic acid (DCA), laetrile, hydrazine sulfate, and cannabis. The shamans of the Amazon and the holy water of Lourdes, France, have also been proclaimed as healers. Some other treatments like cancer vaccines and hyperthermia, photodynamic, and sonodynamic therapy are the subjects of intensive research and have great potential to become conventional treatments for cancer. However, others like Rife machines, ozone therapy, poly-MVA, and Naessens 714X have not received adequate scientific validation.

Some alternative treatments are more useful for symptom control than direct cancer treatment. For example, reiki and acupuncture may be effective for improving cancer patients' quality of life, while therapies like lymphatic massage and hyperbaric oxygen may reduce side effects of cancer treatment. Regardless of the particular therapy or its intended use, the principles guiding the inclusion of any treatment should be (1) to keep an open mind but insist on the clinical evidence of the treatment's benefits, and (2) to "do no harm" by staying clear of treatments like Coley's Toxins, cesium chloride, geranium, and chaparral, all of which have serious potential side effects.

CONCLUSION

By now, it is evident that there many more potential cancer treatments beyond the conventional therapies. A wide range of drugs, vitamins, herbs, supplements, diets, spiritual activities, and other methods may also serve as effective components of a cancer treatment plan, especially when employed in tandem with conventional therapies. As this chapter makes clear, an ideal anti-cancer cocktail has both a conventional and an unconventional dimension, and the various treatments comprising each dimension work via an array of biological mechanisms, some of which overlap. Simply put, all possible and appropriate treatments should be enlisted to fight cancer, provided they are safe and backed by science.

Now that you are familiar with the specific types of treatment cocktail therapy may involve, we can take a look at how to implement this therapy in a step-by-step fashion. Once you understand the process of cocktail therapy and read about potential treatment agents in more detail (see Part 2 on page 85), you can then turn to page 173, which provides case studies demonstrating how this therapy can be carried out in a practical, safe, and effective manner.

6

Putting It All Together

S o far, we have examined the reasons why a multidimensional approach to cancer treatment is superior to the conventional linear strategy, and reviewed the broad scope of conventional and unconventional cancer therapies. Now the key is to put it all together. In this chapter, I suggest five practical considerations for anyone diagnosed with cancer, followed by six principles that should form the basis of an optimal cancer treatment plan. Finally, I lay out the rules for a logical, step-by-step cocktail treatment strategy for cancer.

WHAT TO DO IF YOU ARE DIAGNOSED WITH CANCER

Dealing with cancer is as mentally and emotionally burdensome as it is physically taxing, but there are some practical steps you can take to ensure that you receive the best possible care and achieve an optimal outcome. Highlighted below are the five foremost considerations when seeking ideal cancer care and treatment.

1. Find the Right Doctors

As with any journey or project, the key is to find the best guide or project manager. In this case, you need the best doctor to expertly devise and implement a treatment plan. Not long ago, a Mayo Clinic study identified seven traits—in no particular order—that patients appreciated in their doctors.[1] The study suggested that doctors should be:

- **Confident.** "The doctor's confidence gives me confidence."

- **Empathetic.** "The doctor tries to understand what I am feeling and experiencing, physically and emotionally, and communicates that understanding to me."

- **Humane.** "The doctor is caring, compassionate, and kind."

- **Personal.** "The doctor is interested in me more than just as a patient, interacts with me, and remembers me as an individual."

- **Forthright.** "The doctor tells me what I need to know in plain language and in a forthright manner."

- **Respectful.** "The doctor takes my input seriously and works with me."

- **Thorough.** "The doctor is conscientious and persistent."

This list includes desirable personality traits, but it does not address the importance of the doctor's expertise. Because cancer is such a complex condition, its treatment requires a doctor who is not only kind and understanding, but also knowledgeable. An ideal cancer doctor should thus have superior experience and technical know-how, both in breadth and depth, in order to deal with a particular cancer. Just as important, he or she should be open-minded to new and different treatment options.

2. Obtain Second Opinions

In most instances, and especially for relatively uncommon cancers, it is worth your while to obtain expert second opinions on the cancer diagnosis and treatment plan before settling on one particular doctor or team with which you feel comfortable. People who have been diagnosed with less common cancers (types other than breast, colon, lung, ovary, or prostate) may want to visit a major university hospital or one of the sixty-six cancer centers in the United States as designated by the NCI. (For a full listing, visit www.cancer.gov and search for "Cancer Centers List.") Many patients are surprised by the wide range of options and approaches offered by unaffiliated doctors and institutions. However, it is also important to avoid going overboard when seeking expert advice. In general, there is no need for more than two or three additional opinions. I have seen patients who visited multiple experts only to end up more confused than ever.

3. Choose One Lead Doctor

Sometimes, it is hard to find one doctor who is knowledgeable in all areas. For example, surgeons are more skilled at operating and determining if surgery is warranted in a particular case; radiation doctors obviously know more about radiation techniques; and chemotherapists are more familiar with the latest chemotherapy regimens and their side effects. As such, a team approach is often necessary for a complex condition like cancer. But having a team of specialists and gathering second opinions does *not* mean spreading the responsibility of your care among multiple institutions or doctors. You may end up with a specialist for practically every aspect of your disease, but without one leading physician to oversee your treatment in its entirety and ensure that all of your needs are met. A committee of doctors can provide useful advice and recommendations, but decision-making should be done by one trustworthy doctor, usually a medical oncologist, who will be responsible for and coordinate your overall care.

4. Learn as Much as Possible Yourself

Since information is easily accessible today, you should try to learn as much as possible about your condition and treatment options. Think of it as taking an expedition in unfamiliar terrain. Although you, the traveler, can hire a competent guide, it is certainly helpful to study the map yourself before embarking on the journey. Similarly, the more you understand your disease and treatment options, the more capable you are of asking good questions and making the right decisions with your doctor. But again, do not go overboard reading about your options and then attempting to implement your own treatment. The goal is to be a self-advocate, not to self-treat.

5. Express Yourself

As a patient, it is important for you to think about what you really want or do not want, and tell your doctor upfront. Every person is different and every cancer is different, and this affects the course of treatment. For example, consider the importance of quality of life to you: Do you want to take every possible measure to overcome the disease, or would you rather not sacrifice life quality in a relentless pursuit of treatment efficacy? Are you deathly afraid of chemotherapy or highly sensitive to pharmaceuticals? Do you think diet is very important? Do you want to spend a holiday away with family and thus need some time off from treatment? Do you want to know everything about your disease down to every last detail, including your chances of survival? Alternatively, you may prefer to leave your cancer treatment solely in the hands of your doctor. Whatever your priorities may be, they are important—so you should discuss them with your treating oncologist.

The treatment guidelines discussed so far apply to all cancer patients, and should be considered soon after the diagnosis. Once a program of treatment has been decided, it is time to implement it. Six principles, which are described in the next section, should guide the execution of your treatment plan.

AN OPTIMAL COCKTAIL TREATMENT PLAN

The design plan for constructing a house can be drawn only after architects and contractors are consulted. In the same way, a treatment plan for cancer is devised after a patient has chosen a doctor to be charge of their care, learned as much as possible about their disease and therapy options, and clarified their own goals and desires. Outlined below are six principles that should guide treatment plans for any cancer. It is important that you, the patient, are aware of these principles so that you can continue to ask your doctor good questions and receive the best possible care. Although these principles are discussed with cocktail therapy in mind, they may be followed for conventional cancer therapy as well.

1. Treatments Should Have Clear Goals

Inhibiting cancer development, treating cancer, and preventing cancer recurrence are three different things. Moreover, treatments intended to improve survival differ from treatments intended to allay cancer-related symptoms or enhance quality of life. Therefore, the goal or goals of treatment should be clear at every point in time over the course of therapy.

2. Treatments Should Be Tailored and Targeted

The basic goal of cocktail therapy is to attack the cancer from multiple angles in order to overwhelm it. However, treatment should also be tailored to the patient and the specific biology of the particular cancer. Certain cancers, such as breast and prostate cancer, respond better to hormones, while others, like melanoma and kidney cancer, are more responsive to immunotherapy. There are also some cancers that are not sensitive to radiation, and other types that may not respond to chemotherapy. An optimal treatment cocktail uses different modalities and classes of agents with diverse mechanisms of action, but with the specific biology of the cancer in mind.

Besides taking the cancer's biology into account, it is important to consider the location of the cancer in the body. Different battles are fought in different locales and with different weaponry—battleships are used on the ocean, while fighter jets are used in the sky, for example. Similarly, a different treatment approach may be taken depending on if the cancer involves the brain, liver, lungs, bones, or other area of the body. For instance, aerosolized medicine—medicine administered via a nebulizer or inhaler—may be used for lung cancer, and liver cancers can be treated with a broad range of treatments, including *localized radiation, radiofrequency ablation* (RFA), *microsphere therapy* (specifically SIR-Spheres), and *transarterial chemoembolization*

(TACE). (See the inset on page 20.) As such, a cocktailed approach to any particular cancer may involve tailored biology- and region-specific treatments administered simultaneously in order to yield optimal results.

3. Treatments Should Be Evidence-Based

There are many treatments for cancer, some conventional and some unconventional, some approved and some unapproved, some expensive and some inexpensive. But the bottom line is to use what works. Therefore, individual and combination treatments alike should be judged based on whether or not their effectiveness has been proven. Namely, there should be meaningful and demonstrated evidence of the treatment's efficacy in humans. Treatments that have been tested or found to have an effect only in animals or in test tubes should generally be avoided, especially if they involve potential risks and side effects.

Some new and expensive treatments have caught the attention of both conventional cancer doctors and the public in recent years and, as a result, have become widely prescribed. Unfortunately, the actual benefits of these treatments may be very limited. Take the drug bevacizumab, or Avastin, as an example. An anti-angiogenic medication, Avastin cost $2.25 billion to develop and is now FDA-approved for advanced colon, lung, breast, and brain cancers. With a price tag that averages close to $100,000 per year, Avastin is one of the most popular anti-cancer drugs in the world, and billions of dollars are spent on it annually. But extensive research, FDA approval, a high price tag, and popularity cannot make a drug effective: Studies have shown that Avastin prolongs life by only a few months.

In February 2008, Senator Chuck Grassley asked the US Government Accountability Office (GAO) to look into the FDA's approval of drugs like Avastin, which "appear to have little to no effect in protecting lives and increasing health."[2] In an article entitled "The Evidence Gap," which was printed in *The New York Times* in July 2008, the oncologist and insurance executive Dr. Lee Newcomer said that patients, insurers, and the public, who ultimately foots the bill, were not well-served by Avastin. According to Dr. Newcomer, if a drug stops tumor progression without helping a patient live longer or feel better, then "you're treating an X-ray."[3] Later, in the summer of 2010, Britain's National Institute for Health and Clinical Excellence advised the UK's National Health Service against using Avastin for patients with advanced breast cancer. The Institute called the clinical trial data "disappointing" and the cost "too high for the limited and uncertain benefit it may offer patients." Subsequently, an FDA advisory panel decided in a vote of twelve to one to revoke the agency's approval of the drug for breast cancer.[4]

This example shows why you should not assume that a treatment is effective just because it is approved. Likewise, you should not assume that a statistically effective drug can produce meaningful results. A treatment that extends life for two months is not as meaningful, or significant, as a treatment that extends life for two years. And any drug that extends life but causes debilitating side effects is not as meaningful a treatment as a drug that extends life without negatively impacting life quality. You should always ask your doctor for evidence of a treatment's effectiveness, and inquire about both the potential risks and the side effects.

Many grandiose claims have also been made about the healing power of various herbs and other alternative treatments for cancer. Especially in the current age of Internet marketing, everything from asparagus to zeolite has been touted as a cancer remedy. These claims are often based on studies that are small, biased, poorly conducted, or limited to animals and test tubes, and thus have minimal validity and no realistic implications for human patients. (Dr. Judah Folkman, the founder of angiogenesis, famously remarked, "If you have cancer and are a mouse, we can take good care of you."[5]) Some well-publicized therapies are accompanied by testimonials from those who supposedly benefited, but anecdotes are neither scientific nor completely reliable. Factual accounts are usually the exception rather than the rule.

Still, unconventional treatments usually cost much less and, by and large, have milder or fewer side effects than conventional therapies. Therefore, while not as much evidence is required in order to use them, responsible doctors and rational patients should insist on proof of an alternative treatment's efficacy in humans before prescribing or taking them. See page 107 of Part 2 for a list of alternative treatments that may be effective against cancer.

4. Treatments Should Be Synergistic

A cocktail strategy for cancer involves combining different therapies to produce synergy. Chapter 4 (see page 45) provides a short list of synergistic combinations among conventional treatments, but combinations of unconventional treatments, as well as conventional and unconventional treatments, can work synergistically, as well. Some examples include:

- Heat-based treatments (hyperthermia therapy) with chemotherapy[6] and radiation.[7]

- Individual herbal ingredients such as turmeric (curcumin) with chemotherapy,[8] or green tea polyphenol EGCG with targeted therapy.[9]

- Supplements, such as melatonin, with chemotherapy,[10] or gamma-linolenic acid (GLA) with hormone therapy.[11]

- Traditional Chinese herbal formulas with chemotherapy and radiation.[12]

- Various herbal combinations, such as PC-SPES.[13]

- Vitamin K_3 and vitamin C.[14]

- Vitamins, such as vitamin D, with chemotherapy[15] and immunotherapy.[16]

In sum, the core principle underlying the cocktail approach is the use of more than one effective treatment at a time in order to enhance the results. As the law of additive advantage states, one plus one equals two. But one of the keys to superior cocktail therapy is the use of conventional and unconventional agents that can work together synergistically, enhancing the treatments' beneficial effects so that one plus one is *greater than* two.

5. Treatments Should Not Be Potentially Antagonistic

This is the opposite of the previous principle. Obviously, using treatments that might cancel out effects of one another or enhance each other's toxicity is undesirable. While many conventional treatments used in combination may enhance each another, full-dose radiation and chemotherapy may produce intolerable toxicity when combined. It is for this reason that these treatments must be administered sequentially in the majority of cases.

By and large, potential negative interactions between conventional modalities and drugs are well known, and clinicians are careful to avoid such unwarranted combinations. However, potential negative interactions between conventional and unconventional treatments should be highlighted, since they are not as well known. For example, estrogen- and hormone-stimulating herbs and supplements—ginseng, soy, licorice, red clover, dong quai—may reduce the effectiveness of anti-estrogen therapy, which is often used for estrogen-positive breast and ovarian cancer, as well as promote the growth of hormonally sensitive cancer cells. In addition, antioxidants such as vitamins C and E may diminish the beneficial effects of conventional cytotoxic therapy, which include chemotherapies like cyclophosphamide and anthracyclines.

Clinical experience with such potential interactions is limited, however, and some studies even suggest that the concerns may not be warranted in all circumstances. For instance, estrogenic soy may actually protect against estrogen-sensitive breast cancer,[17] and antioxidants CoQ_{10}[18] and melatonin[19] have proven beneficial when applied in tandem with chemotherapy. Nevertheless, this is an area of ongoing controversy, and it is better to be prudent and stay away from risk and controversy where it exists.

6. Treatments Should Take Life Quality Into Account

A good doctor treats not only the cancer, but also the patient. Patients who suffer from the disease or the toxic effects from treatment have concerns about quality-of-life issues such as depression, nausea and loss of appetite, sexual dysfunction, and general weakness and fatigue. All of these issues need to be considered when planning a course of treatment, which all too often sacrifices quality of life in favor of survival time. But it is just as important to live *well* as it is to live *long*. In this regard, physicians should be sensitive to your concerns and, at the same time, you should be assertive in voicing your concerns and priorities.

One particular case in my own practice comes to mind. An eighty-two-year-old jazz musician with prostate cancer came to me insisting that he did not want surgery, radiation, or hormone therapy as conventional cancer doctors had recommended. He told me point-blank that he had recently married a young woman and wanted to live out his remaining years in a fulfilling manner rather than risk impotency due to treatment. I respected his concerns and treated him with common off-label drugs, herbs, vitamins, and a low-fat diet. Now in his nineties, he is well and, in fact, just recently remarried.

Increasingly, clinical trials of cancer treatments are going beyond measuring the effectiveness of treatment, and assessing how the treatments affect quality of life as well. In addition, many hospitals have instituted palliative care teams to help cancer patients with symptom management. The Dana-Farber Cancer Institute at Harvard University even has a Quality of Life Clinic. Although extended survival does not necessarily translate to better life quality, the latest research involving over 10,000 patients from the Mayo Clinic[20] in the United States and the European Organization for Research and Treatment of Cancer (EORTC)[21] shows that better quality of life is actually correlated with improved survival. This is all the more reason to take quality-of-life issues seriously.

Cancer, in all of its many forms, can cause pain and suffering as intense as any human affliction, and many cancer treatments cause intense side effects that compound a patient's misery. In any treatment program, the quality of survival deserves as much attention as survival itself.

DESIGNING A TREATMENT COCKTAIL

Once a doctor or medical team has been assembled and a treatment plan determined, cocktail therapy can be implemented. Step-by-step guidelines are provided in the pages that follow, and they should be carefully considered before putting the cocktail strategy into action. However, this is *not* a do-it-yourself menu. The guidelines presented below are meant to serve as a kind of "map" that an amateur hiker or sailor would take with him on a challenging journey: The map is not intended to replace a professional guide or boat captain, but rather to function as a tool, familiarizing the hiker with the terrain, enhancing the teamwork of the hiker and guide, and making the journey an overall better experience. In the same way, the guidelines provided here are meant to familiarize you with the details of treatment cocktails so that you can meaningfully assess and make intelligent decisions about your course of cancer treatment, as well as effectively communicate with your doctors.

Step 1: Use Conventional Medicine as a Backbone

Classical treatments like surgery, chemotherapy, and radiation should be the foundation of any cancer treatment plan, along with modern conventional treatments such as targeted therapy, anti-angiogenic therapy, immunotherapy, and other new approaches. Although these therapies have potential side effects, they also have well-defined outcomes as evidenced by formal clinical trials and FDA approval. The conventional treatments should then be complemented by and combined with unconventional treatments in order to reduce side effects and/or improve the outcome. Therefore, if cancer is localized to one area of the body and can be easily removed, surgery should be performed. In addition, if chemotherapy or radiation can meaningfully improve the treatment outcome, extend survival time, or reduce the risk of recurrence, it should be seriously considered as long as its potential negative impact on life quality is tolerable and acceptable. Only rarely should conventional approaches be left out, such as when they may seriously compromise life quality or will not meaningfully improve the outcome. However, this decision should be made on a personalized basis and discussed with a doctor in depth.

The emphasis on conventional treatments is important. Embracing unconventional treatments like herbs, vitamins, and off-label drugs does not mean forsaking surgery or chemotherapy. This book does not endorse only alternative cancer treatment, but rather the integrative and complementary use of non-standard approaches. To use an analogy, consider how school grades and test scores often serve as the backbone of a college application. Grades and test scores are usually necessary, and to base college admission on extracurricular activities would be unsound, if not unrealistic, for most students. Unconventional therapies are the equivalent of extracurricular activities: They can make or break the "application," but they cannot replace good grades and test scores.

Step 2: Add Unconventional Treatments

After the "backbone" treatments have been determined, unconventional therapies can be added, either simultaneously or sequentially, in order to reduce side effects and/or enhance the effectiveness of the foundational treatments. (These unconventional therapies can also serve as backups when the conventional treatments do not work or if they are not being used at all due to the patient's preferences, intolerable side effects, or because they previously failed.) For example, off-label drugs, vitamins, and supplements may be used to reduce the risk of breast cancer recurrence after a patient undergoes standard surgery, chemotherapy, and radiation. Alternatively, off-label drugs, vitamins, and supplements can be taken alongside the conventional treatment in order to diminish side effects or improve its efficacy. Of course, unconventional therapies should always be considered for those patients who refuse or cannot tolerate conventional treatment.

Step 3: Carry Out the Plan in Steps

With a cocktail regimen, it is not necessary to know what particular treatment is working as long as the cocktail is effective, as opposed to a clinical trial setting where the goal is to learn precisely what works and what does not. At the same time, however, doctors still want to know what causes a certain side effect if one should occur. This is why taking a step-by-step approach to cocktail treatment is important—it better enables doctors to identify the cause of a problem if something goes wrong. For example, if off-label drugs, vitamins, and Chinese herbs are to be taken at the same time as chemotherapy, each group should be added separately. This way, if undesirable side effects or interactions occur, or if an allergy develops, the root of the problem can be more easily identified.

In general, you and your doctor should first decide on a conventional treatment program. Then, off-label drugs can be incorporated followed by herbs, vitamins, other supplements, and specialized diets or mind-body approaches—in that order. This is like choosing a meal entrée before deciding on side dishes and wine pairings. The logic here is to first apply the treatments most likely to be toxic (usually the "backbone" treatment), followed by less toxic agents. Arguably, the reverse may also be carried out; milder therapies with the least amount of side effects and interaction concerns can be used first—diet, vitamins, supplements, herbs—followed by off-label drugs. It is much more common to implement the most toxic treatments first, but the actual order and sequence of treatment, as well as the time separating the addition of each therapy, may depend on the treatment purpose and the urgency of the situation.

CONCLUSION

Previous chapters examined the reasons why a multidimensional cocktail approach to a complex disease like cancer is superior to the simplistic strategy generally followed in conventional medicine. Standard treatments should be combined more often and, in addition, conventional and unconventional therapies should be used simultaneously to make for a more effective and less toxic treatment regimen. This chapter reviewed the guidelines and other practical considerations for doctors and patients alike when planning such a course of treatment. The advice contained in these pages—from choosing a doctor to clarifying treatment priorities and goals—will enable you, the patient, to have an informed, meaningful discussion with your doctor. Additionally, the principles of cocktail treatment, both theoretical and practical, serve as a useful reference not only for physicians, but also for patients and their families so that they can become their own advocates and more involved in the treatment process.

Now you should know about some substances, from pharmaceutical drugs to medicinal herbs, that may have useful anti-cancer potential. Part 2 lists a number of off-label drugs and dietary supplements that may be effective for cancer treatment and, therefore, might be included in an anti-cancer cocktail. The decision to take any particular substance should be guided by a knowledgeable and experienced healthcare professional, and the information contained in Part 2 should be discussed with your doctor. Once you have familiarized yourself with these alternative and complementary treatments, you can then turn to page 173 for three case studies that illustrate real-life applications of anti-cancer cocktail therapy.

Off-Label Drugs and Dietary Supplements Lists

Off-Label Drugs

The following pages contain a list of pharmaceutical drugs for which there is published clinical evidence of potential effectiveness against cancer. These drugs are referred to as *off-label* cancer drugs because they have not been specifically approved by the FDA for use against the disease. Rather, they are intended and approved for other medical indications ranging from cough to osteoporosis, and they work via different biological mechanisms. Some of the drugs are even cytotoxic, inducing cancer cell death. Most of the pharmaceuticals included on this list require a prescription, while a few are available over the counter. Still, the use of any pharmaceutical drug—whether prescribed or over-the-counter—should always be carefully monitored by a qualified physician and made known to the primary oncologist. For this reason, no dosage guidelines will be provided here. Patients should follow the directions of the physician who is responsible for their care, and inquire about possible side effects and interactions.

The drugs mentioned in this section are referred to by their generic names, but their US brand names are provided in parentheses. (It is important to note that drugs may be marketed under different names in non-US markets.) This list is by no means exhaustive—there are a number of potentially useful agents in each of the specified drug categories that are not mentioned. Instead, the list identifies commonly used pharmaceuticals that have demonstrable usefulness for cancer treatment and/or prevention. Although the anti-cancer potential of many agents has been studied in the laboratory and animals, the focus here is on the published evidence of their clinical effectiveness, i.e., their efficacy in humans.

ANTACIDS

Antacids are primarily used to treat excessive stomach acid but can also alleviate peptic ulcers, heartburn, acid reflux, and gastro-esophageal reflux disease (GERD). A common antacid is cimetidine (Tagamet), an over-the-counter antihistamine stomach-acid inhibitor that was introduced as a prescription drug for heartburn and ulcers in the 1970s. It went on to become the first drug to bring in a billion US dollars per year in revenue. Cimetidine is a particularly interesting pharmaceutical, having been studied as an off-label treatment for a wide range of conditions from fibromyalgia to warts. More significant is the drug's many anti-cancer properties, making it a perfect example of a safe, inexpensive, and well-evidenced off-label cancer treatment. According to laboratory and animal studies, cimetidine boosts the immune system, inhibits cancer cells, acts as an anti-angiogenic agent, and works synergistically with chemotherapy.

The potential anti-cancer effects of the drug were first discovered in 1979—the same year in which it became FDA approved. Drs. Armitage and Sidner reported the successful use of cimetidine to treat a male patient with head and neck cancer suspected to have spread to his lungs. The patient refused to undergo chemotherapy, but he continued to take cimetidine to treat his upset stomach. After two years on the drug, the cancer had disappeared. A female patient with lung cancer that had spread to her brain also seemed to benefit from cimetidine, which she had been prescribed for heartburn. Her cancer was also reduced in size. However, Drs. Armitage and Sidner could not explain how or why the drug could help fight cancer.[1]

Subsequently, several cases of metastatic melanoma reportedly responded to cimetidine without additional treatment. For some patients, taking the drug even resulted in cancer remission. According to studies, esophageal, stomach, liver, ovarian, kidney, and gallbladder cancer also responded positively to cimetidine. Then, in 1995, Dr. Lars B. Svendsen and his colleagues were among the first to report that cimetidine could improve colon cancer patients' chances of survival. In the same year, a trial found a 36-percent response rate among patients receiving a combination treatment of chemotherapy and cimetidine for metastatic colon cancer. (In contrast, there was a 0-percent response rate among patients receiving only chemotherapy.) The same team also conducted a study showing that 800-milligram doses of the drug taken twice daily for five days leading up to surgery positively affected cancer survival. In Japan, cimetidine was clinically tested for colorectal cancer in a trial that treated patients with daily 800-milligram doses of the drug for one year. As a result, the survival rate among these patients increased from 49.8 percent to 68.8 percent.

Cimetidine is safe and available over the counter, but may produce side effects. It can also raise estrogen levels and, therefore, should be used with caution by women who have breast or gynecologic cancers. Patients should take this drug only as directed by their doctors.

ANTI-ASTHMATICS

Marketed under several brand names, the anti-asthmatic theophylline (TheoDur, Slo-Bid, Quibron, etc.) is an old drug that is chemically similar to caffeine, and typically used to treat respiratory conditions such as asthma and chronic obstructive pulmonary disease. For cancer, the drug is mainly effective for the treatment of lymphoma and leukemia, particularly chronic lymphocytic leukemia (CLL), an incurable form of the disease.

Although there was much laboratory- and animal-based research on theophylline and leukemia prior to the 1990s, the drug's ability to induce apoptosis in leukemic cells was finally demonstrated in humans in 1995.[2] Dr. Frank Mentz and his colleagues reported a case of one leukemia patient who took theophylline for asthma and remained stable for ten years. Since then, there have been other reported cases of CLL patients who responded well to theophylline. In addition, there have been trials of the drug as both a single-agent treatment and an adjunctive treatment used in combination with chemotherapy. One trial found that 76 percent of CLL patients treated with only theophylline remained stable,[3] and another showed that treatment regimens including the drug worked effectively for patients with relapsed CLL, as well as non-Hodgkin's lymphomas.[4]

The doses of theophylline used in these trials were as low as 200 milligrams, taken twice per day. The patients who participated in the trials seemed to tolerate this amount, but theophylline may produce side effects and drug interactions. Therefore, its use should always be prescribed and closely monitored by a healthcare professional, and patients should take the drug only as directed.

ANTIBIOTICS

Antibiotics are substances usually derived from a mold or bacterium, and used to kill microorganisms and cure infections. Interestingly, some chemotherapies are related to antibiotics, so it is not a coincidence that certain chemotherapy drugs—such as doxorubicin (Adriamycin) and mitomycin (Mutamycin)—have names similar to that of antibiotics, like erythromycin and clindamycin. The fact that some common antibiotics have anti-cancer potential, therefore, is not completely surprising. Prime examples include *macrolide antibiotics* such as clarithromycin, which may be effective in cases of multiple myeloma and non-small cell lung cancer, as well as *quinolone antibiotics* like ciprofloxacin, which may be useful for bladder cancer.

Clarithromycin (Biaxin) is an antibiotic commonly prescribed for respiratory, skin, ear, nose, and throat infections. Its anti-cancer potential was first reported in 1999[5] and, since then, has been extensively studied in conventional oncology, especially for use against myeloma. Doses of 500 milligrams taken twice daily—the amount normally used to treat infections—have been used with the anti-cancer drugs thalidomide and dexamethasone in a combination regimen known as "BLT-D." The combination was found to be highly effective for patients with both myeloma and *Waldenström's macroglobulinemia*, a rare type of non-Hodgkin's lymphoma.[6] A more recent trial involved administering another combination treatment known as "BiRD"—clarithromycin (Biaxin), lenalidomide (Revlimid), and dexamethasone— to myeloma patients who had not previously received treatment. Overall, 90.3 percent of the patients responded positively to this regimen, and 38.9 percent of patients went into remission.[7] When these patients were compared with those who had not been treated with clarithromycin, it was clear that the antibiotic had significantly influenced the outcome.[8]

Studies of clarithromycin, most of which have been conducted and published in Japan, have shown that the drug is effective for not only less common blood cancers but also the much more common non-small-cell lung cancer. A controlled clinical trial showed that clarithromycin doubled the survival time of advanced non-small-cell lung cancer patients and produced only minor side effects.[9]

Another family of antibiotics that may be useful for cancer treatment is quinolone antibiotics, particularly ciprofloxacin (Cipro). As early as 1992, ciprofloxacin was found to inhibit bladder cancer and, in 1999, Dr. Donald Lamm and his colleagues suggested that it may reduce bladder cancer recurrence as well.[10] Unfortunately, there have not have been any trials organized to test this hypothesis.

Other common antibiotics such as tetracyclines may also be effective cancer treatment, which is a possibility waiting to be explored. Patients should speak to their medical provider before taking any of these antibiotics for cancer, as side effects and drug interactions are possible. The drugs should be used only as directed.

ANTICOAGULANTS

The relationship between cancer and blood clotting has been known since the mid-nineteenth century. Since then, the link between the blood-clotting system and the formation and spread of tumors has been confirmed in a number of laboratory and animal studies. It may not come as a surprise, then, that a wide range of *anticoagulants*— anti-clotting medications that thin the blood via various biological mechanisms—also inhibit cancer. There are two groups of drugs that thin the blood or affect blood clotting. First, there are antiplatelet agents such as dipyridamole, which are members of the anti-inflammatory drug class (see page 94 for more about anti-inflammatory drugs). The focus of this section, however, is the second group of anti-coagulants—drugs of the warfarin and heparin families. These drugs affect blood clotting in ways independent of platelet function.

Warfarin (Coumadin) is a synthetic chemical that was initially used as rat poison and later approved to prevent and dissolve blood clots. Over the years, studies have shown that adding warfarin to treatment regimens for certain types of cancer may be beneficial. We now know, for example, that prolonged warfarin usage may decrease the risk of prostate cancer,[11] as well as improve survival for patients with extensive small-cell lung cancer.[12]

The other major anticoagulant drug is *heparin,* which is naturally isolated from animal liver (*hepar* is the Greek word for liver) and one of the oldest drugs still in use. *Low molecular weight heparins* (LMWH) are modern pharmacological derivatives of natural heparin, and are less toxic and easier to use. LMWHs, such as enoxaparin (Lovenox) and dalteparin (Fragmin), are safer and more effective than vitamin-K antagonists like warfarin for improving cancer survival.

There is quite a bit of laboratory- and animal-based evidence demonstrating heparin's various anti-cancer activities, which include reducing the ability of cancer cells to stick together and form tumors, as well as inhibiting proliferation.[13] In cancer patients, particularly those with advanced pancreatic cancer, LMWHs used in conjunction with chemotherapy may offer significant advantages in terms of survival.[14] According to a recent scientific review, heparin also improves survival for cancer patients in general, especially patients with limited small-cell lung cancer. In addition, the drug may be very beneficial for patients with cancer that has not significantly spread or with a longer life expectancy.[15]

Although the benefits of warfarin and heparin are well documented for certain types of cancer, they may pose side effects such as increased risk of bleeding. Using these drugs also comes with some minor inconveniences, such as injections (heparin) and frequent blood tests to prevent overdosing (warfarin). Patients should carefully weigh the risks and benefits of the drugs before taking them, consult a healthcare professional experienced in their usage, and use them only as directed.

See also Anti-inflammatory Drugs and Antiplatelet Drugs.

ANTIDEPRESSANTS

It goes without saying that cancer patients may experience depression after being diagnosed, and thus may be prescribed an antidepressant. But the beneficial effects of antidepressants may go beyond mood improvement for those with cancer, as research indicates that antidepressant drugs have the ability to kill brain cancer cells in the test tube. Recently, British doctors tested the effectiveness of the antidepressant clomipramine (Anafranil) when used as an adjunctive treatment for brain cancer. Clomipramine, a medication that belongs to an old class of antidepressants known as *tricyclics*, was given to twenty-seven brain cancer patients, 80 percent of whom showed a reduction in their cancer following the treatment.[16] Other antidepressants have also been found to contain anti-cancer properties in laboratory testing. The usefulness of these drugs, which include the more modern selective serotonin-reuptake inhibitors (SSRIs) like paroxetine (Paxil) and fluoxetine (Prozac), may extend to other cancers.[17]

Antidepressants require a prescription, so their use should be discussed with a qualified physician. Patients should also consider the potential risks and side effects before using an antidepressant, and take them only as directed.

ANTI-DIABETICS

Used to treat diabetes by lowering blood sugar concentration, antidiabetic drugs may serve as potential off-label treatments for cancer, especially the medications designed to enhance insulin sensitivity. Such drugs include *peroxisome proliferator-activated receptor (PPAR) modulators,* like rosiglitazone (Avandia) and pioglitazone (Actos), and *biguanides,* such as metformin (Glucophage).

PPARs, a group of proteins that regulate gene expression, play a key role in cell metabolism and growth. PPAR modulators are drugs that act upon PPARs, and their anti-cancer effects have been repeatedly demonstrated for a wide range of cancers in both animals and the laboratory. In humans, one study found that patients with advanced differentiated thyroid cancer remained stable for an extended period of time after receiving rosiglitazone (Avandia) treatment. Researchers at the University of California at San Francisco found that 40 percent of thyroid cancer patients treated with the drug either stabilized or experienced tumor shrinkage.[18] In addition, German medical scientists studied the effects of PPAR modulators taken in conjunction COX-2 inhibitors and low-dose chemotherapy, discovering that this combination was somewhat effective for people with recurrent brain cancer.[19]

PPAR modulators should be taken only under the supervision of a doctor, as they can cause undesirable side effects like fluid retention. There has been concern regarding the safety of some PPAR-modulating drugs, and some countries have removed them from the market altogether. Rosiglitazone, for instance, may increase the risk of heart attack and even cause bladder cancer after prolonged use. For this reason, PPAR modulators are currently undergoing review by the FDA to ensure their safety. Patients should absolutely not take such drugs unless prescribed by a qualified physician who has carefully weighed the potential risks and benefits. Moreover, safer PPAR-modulators like pioglitazone—which does not seem to pose the risks associated with rosiglitazone—should generally not be prescribed for more than twenty-four months for safety reasons. In the meantime, we must await a new generation of PPAR-modulating drugs that lack cardiac and bladder cancer risks.

The other type of anti-diabetic medication with anti-cancer potential is a biguanide called metformin (Glucophage), which originates from the French Lilac (*Galega officinalis*) plant. First described in 1957, metformin is one of the safest and most commonly prescribed drugs for diabetes around the world. Its biological actions, which involve sugar metabolism, include suppressing the liver's sugar production, increasing insulin sensitivity, and decreasing the absorption of sugar in the intestines. Scientists have been uncovering the roles that sugar metabolism and insulin signaling play in cancer growth,[20] and there is now ample laboratory research showing that metformin may be effective against the disease. A study from the University of Dundee in 2009, which involved 4,085 patients, suggested that people who take metformin for more than ten years may boost their protection against all forms of cancer by 30 to 40 percent.[21] Also in 2009, Dr. Gonzalez-Angulo and a team at MD Anderson Cancer Center studied 2,529 early-stage breast cancer patients who underwent chemotherapy, and found that the treatment response rate among those who took metformin was three times higher than the rate among those who had not taken the drug.[22] This result, according to Dr. Gonzalez-Angulo, is probably due to decreased insulin levels among those who took metformin, since insulin is a known growth factor for cancer. More studies investigating this connection are currently being organized.

Metformin is a relatively benign drug and, therefore, produces very few side effects. For most cancer patients, the drug can be safely taken as an off-label adjunctive treatment. However, patients should always err on the side of caution and consult their medical provider before taking metformin, as it may interact with various medications.

ANTIFUNGALS

Available both over the counter and by prescription, antifungal drugs are used to treat topical and systemic fungal infections. Recent studies also suggest that some antifungal medications may be used as anti-cancer agents. One such medication is ketoconazole (Nizoral), which treats athlete's foot, ringworm, *Candida* (yeast infection), and jock itch. It is also an ingredient used in anti-dandruff shampoos. In addition to its antifungal actions, ketoconazole is an anti-hormone that specifically targets male hormones. This action suggests that the drug may be effective for hormonally driven prostate cancer.[23]

A study from UCLA in 2005 found that a high percentage of prostate cancer patients responded positively to ketoconazole-based therapy, even though standard hormone therapy had been ineffective.[24] Trials of ketoconazole used in combination with chemotherapy are currently underway. Additionally, other antifungal medicines, such as clotrimazole, are being investigated as potential cancer treatments. Antifungal medications may have side effects and should be taken only as directed by a physician.

ANTI-INFLAMMATORY DRUGS

Anti-inflammatory drugs are arguably the most commonly used medications in the world. They are primarily taken to relieve fever and mild to moderate pain, and to reduce the body's inflammatory response to infection or physical trauma. Included in this category are *nonsteroidal anti-inflammatory drugs* (NSAIDs)—aspirin, ibuprofen (Motrin, Advil), and naprosyn (Aleve), for example—and drugs derived from NSAIDs called *cyclooxygenase-2 (COX-2) inhibitors,* such as celecoxib (Celebrex). Each of these groups is discussed separately below.

Traditional NSAIDs

Mainly used to treat pain and fever, NSAIDs also act as antiplatelet agents and, therefore, can prevent heart attacks and strokes. The original and prototypical NSAID is aspirin, which is derived from the bark of willow trees. Forty thousand tons of aspirin are produced and consumed annually worldwide.

Although the drug has been in existence for more than a century, aspirin's anti-cancer potential was not proposed until the 1970s, and its effectiveness as a cancer preventative was confirmed only in the 1990s. Its role in reducing the incidence of many types of cancer has been widely studied, with the most encouraging results for colon and breast cancer. Regular use of aspirin for at least five years has been shown to lower the risk of colorectal cancer by 20 percent or more.[25] More significant, perhaps, is that aspirin use has been associated with improved survival rates for breast cancer patients, as well as reduced recurrence of the disease. A recent analysis of data from a large Harvard study (Nurses' Health Study), which followed 4,614 female nurses with breast cancer, found that the women who took aspirin decreased their risk of metastases and death by nearly 50 percent.[26] A smaller and earlier Harvard study reported similar results: Survival rates improved among colon cancer patients who took aspirin.[27] The drug may also be effective in the treatment of esophageal, gastric, lung, and ovarian cancers.

Although relatively safe and available over the counter, aspirin has been known to thin the blood, increase the risk of bleeding, and cause ulcers. Other adverse side effects are also possible, so patients should consult a healthcare professional before using aspirin and take the drug only as directed.

COX-2 Inhibitors

COX-2 inhibitors belong to the NSAID family, but specifically target the COX-2 enzyme, which is responsible for pain and inflammation. This enzyme is active in many cancers and, therefore, a desirable target for cancer treatment and prevention. COX-2 inhibitors have been intensively studied in animals and the laboratory, and have been shown to hinder not only angiogenesis but also the proliferation and metastasis of cancer cells. In addition, COX-2 inhibitors may prevent precancerous growths and reduce cancer occurrence.

In 1999, the FDA approved the COX-2 inhibitor celecoxib (Celebrex) for the preventative treatment of precancerous intestinal polyps known as *adenomas*. These polyps are often caused by a hereditary condition known as *familial adenomatous polyposis,* which may lead to colon cancer. A landmark trial in 2006, which studied more than 2,000 patients with this condition, found that those who took celecoxib developed 33 to 45 percent fewer adenomas.[28] Moreover, population-based research has demonstrated that the daily use of a COX-2 inhibitor significantly reduces the risk of breast, colon, lung, and prostate cancer.[29]

The effectiveness of COX-2 inhibitors used as both a single-agent treatment and in combination with conventional cancer therapies is currently being explored. In 2010 alone, the National Cancer Institute sponsored thirty-five clinical trials involving COX-2 inhibitors, and encouraging results have been reported. A trial conducted at Cornell University found that celecoxib (400 milligrams twice a day) combined with chemotherapy was effective for 65 percent of the patients who participated—a significantly higher response rate than that of chemotherapy alone. Additionally, in one-third of the patients, tumors were reduced by 95 percent. By comparison, such dramatic improvement had occurred in only 6 percent of patients previously.[30]

A separate trial found that celecoxib enhanced hormone therapy for patients with advanced breast cancer.[31]

Although there is demonstrable evidence that COX-2 inhibitors are useful for cancer prevention and treatment, the drug rofecoxib (Vioxx), was removed from the market in September 2004 due to concerns that it increased the risk of heart attack and stroke. This was a temporary roadblock to the further development of these drugs as treatment for cancer, but the search is on once again for newer and safer COX-2 inhibitors.

Celecoxib is relatively safe but requires a prescription. Patients should consult a healthcare professional before using the drug and take it only as directed.

ANTIMALARIALS

As their name suggests, antimalarial medications are used to treat *malaria,* a mosquito-borne infectious disease caused by the *Plasmodium* family of parasites. A common antimalarial drug is chloroquine (Aralen), an inexpensive, relatively benign, and widely available medication introduced in 1947. Today, the drug is also occasionally used to treat conditions such as arthritis and lupus, and there is evidence that it may be effective for cancer treatment as well. Some of chloroquine's better known effects are *radiosensitization* and *chemosensitization,* which means that it enhances the responsiveness of cancer cells to radiation and chemotherapy. Recent studies on brain cancer have found that 150-milligram doses of the drug per day, in combination with conventional radiation and chemotherapy, may more than double survival time.[32]

Another antimalarial with anti-cancer potential is artesunate, a semi-synthetic drug derived from the *Artemisia* plant, also known as Qing Hao or sweet wormwood. The mother compound of artesunate is artemisinin, which exerts not only antimalarial effects but also anti-tumor activity via multiple mechanisms, including cytotoxicity, anti-angiogenesis, and apoptosis. Artesunate may be effective for melanoma in particular; one patient treated with the drug was still alive forty-seven months after being diagnosed with stage IV uveal melanoma, the prognosis for which is two to five months.[33] The effectiveness of artesunate has also been tested on advanced lung cancer patients in a recent trial, in which it was combined with chemotherapy. The short-term survival rate among the participating patients improved, and no additional side effects were reported.[34] My group at the nonprofit Institute of East-West Medicine, with support from the Gray Charitable Trust and others, is now actively studying the anti-cancer potential of antimalarial drugs.

Both chloroquine and artesunate are relatively safe drugs. Chloroquine can be obtained with a prescription, but in the United States, artesunate is available only to patients who have a documented case of severe malaria. Patients must discuss the potential risks and side effects with their medical provider before using these drugs and take them only as directed.

ANTIPLATELET DRUGS

Antiplatelet drugs are pharmaceuticals that decrease platelet stickiness in the blood in order to prevent clotting and, therefore, conditions such as stroke and heart attack. Some classic antiplatelet agents include aspirin (see page 94) and dipyridamole (Persantine), an inexpensive and low-toxicity drug used mainly to prevent recurrent heart attacks and strokes, as well as blood clots associated with artificial heart valves. The drug also has off-label uses from arthritis relief to the treatment of mental disorders like schizophrenia. Given the fact that blood-thinning agents (anticoagulants) may reduce cancer risk and improve survival (see page 89), it is not surprising that medical scientists have looked into the cancer-fighting potential of antiplatelet agents like dipyridamole as well.

The anti-cancer potential of antiplatelet drugs was originally proposed in 1958, but it was in 1987 when a study first produced solid evidence of dipyridamole's cancer-fighting effects. The European Stroke Prevention Study found that taking the drug in combination with aspirin not only cut patients' risk of death due to stroke and heart attack, but also decreased the cancer mortality rate by 30 percent.[35] At the time, scientists believed that dipyridamole inhibited cancer cells from sticking to tissues, in turn preventing the cancer's spread. But since then, they have discovered that the drug may also boost the effectiveness of specific chemotherapy agents (cisplatinum, doxorubicin, etoposide, fluorouracil, methotrexate, vinblastine, etc.) by disabling the ability of cancer cells to expel drugs directed at them. Because dipyridamole may increase the sensitivity of some cancers to chemotherapy, the drug is currently listed on the National Cancer Institute website as a chemo-enhancing agent.

For decades, medical scientists have explored the use of dipyridamole for specific types of cancer. In the 1970s, the British doctor E.H. Rhodes treated melanoma patients with the drug over an eleven-year period and reported a five-year survival rate of 74 percent, which was more than twice the normal rate of 32 percent.[36] Dr. Rhodes believed that dipyridamole could be used to treat other cancers as well, and a Japanese study on advanced gastric cancer later supported his hypothesis. The Japanese researchers found that combining chemotherapy with daily doses of the drug at 4 milligrams per kilogram of body weight (mg/kg) appeared to be effective, safe, and tolerated well by patients.[37]

Furthermore, researchers at UCLA reported a 39-percent response rate among pancreatic cancer patients who were treated with chemotherapy and dipyridamole, and a one-year survival rate of 70 percent. Remarkably, 27 percent of these patients, who initially had inoperable cancer, were able to undergo surgery following the treatment. The one-year survival rate among this group was 83 percent, with one patient still alive four years later.[38] A Japanese team modified the UCLA protocol for their own study, which also reported an 83-percent response rate. This time, 60 percent of patients were able to undergo curative surgery.[39]

The only serious side effect of dipyridamole is an increased risk of bleeding, particularly when the drug is taken in combination with anticoagulants. As with all prescription medications, patients should speak to a healthcare professional about the potential risks, interactions, and side effects. Patients should also follow the directions of their medical provider.

See also Anticoagulants.

ANTI-SEIZURE DRUGS

Also known as antiepileptic drugs, anti-seizure medications act upon the central nervous system and are typically used to treat epilepsy, as well as some mental disorders. One type of anti-seizure agent is valproic acid (Depakote), a short-chain fatty acid (2-propylpetanoic acid) approved for treating epilepsy, migraine headaches, bipolar disorder, and schizophrenia. The drug may also have anti-cancer properties due to its action as a histone deacetylase (HDAC) inhibitor, a class of compounds that have been shown to work against certain cancers. Since 1999, the anti-cancer properties of valproic acid have been explored in clinical trials, with a special focus on leukemias and solid tumors. Researchers have observed a treatment response rate of up to 52 percent in patients with a pre-leukemic condition called *myelodysplastic syndrome*.[40] The drug has also demonstrated some potential against prostate cancer and brain cancer. And according to a 2011 study, valproic acid is associated with a significant increase in survival time for brain cancer patients.[41] A similar medication that has demonstrated anti-cancer potential is levetiracetam (Keppra). This drug may be useful for brain cancer, as it has been shown to increase the sensitivity of brain tumor cells to chemotherapy.[42]

Patients should discuss the possible risks, interactions, and side effects of valproic acid, as well as other anti-seizure drugs, with their medical provider. These drugs should be used only as directed.

ANTITUSSIVES

Antitussive is the official medical term for cough medicine, which is available over the counter and by prescription. A cough suppressant that has been studied as an off-label cancer treatment is noscapine, a non-narcotic compound found in the poppy plant. Although it is not sold in the United States, noscapine is safe, inexpensive, and commonly used in cough medicines in other countries. So far, laboratory and animal research at Emory University in Atlanta, Georgia, has found that the drug can inhibit cancer at doses that produce little toxicity.[43] A clinical trial of noscapine for lymphoma and leukemia was planned for 2003, but terminated early due to apparent funding issues. Trials of the drug for use against prostate cancer and myeloma have been planned, and hopefully, more potent derivatives and analogs of noscapine will be developed in the near future.

BISPHOSPHONATES

Bisphosphonates are a class of drugs used to prevent bone loss and treat osteoporosis. They include the medications alendronate (Fosamax), risedronate (Actonel), and ibandronate (Boniva). Some bisphosphonates, like pamidronate (Aredia) and zoledronate (Zometa), are now being used in cancer management. This use is not considered off-label, since bisphosphonates are often employed when treating cancers that have spread to the bones. Drugs in this class can also have palliative benefits, such as improved quality of life and fewer complications of the disease.

The scientific understanding of bisphosphonates has evolved over the years. In addition to their bone-fortifying effects, the drugs also take direct anti-cancer action. The new generation of bisphosphonate drugs can induce apoptosis and anti-angiogenesis, as well as enhance immunity. It has also been reported that bisphosphonates work synergistically with a broad spectrum of cancer treatments, including COX-2 inhibitors, histone deacetylase (HDAC) inhibitors, immunotherapy (interferon and interleukin), thalidomide (a drug used in the treatment of multiple myeloma), certain chemotherapy drugs, and various targeted therapies.

Certain bisphosphonates in US and non-US markets alike have already been the subjects of studies assessing their effectiveness as potential cancer treatments. Clodronate, an oral bisphosphonate approved for use in Europe and Canada, has been tested on humans, and scientists were encouraged by the results. In 1998, *The New England Journal of Medicine* published a German study in which oral clodronate reduced breast cancer metastases by 50 percent and lowered the risk of death.[44] A randomized, double-blind, controlled study of more than 1,000 patients confirmed these findings in 2006.[45]

Bisphosphonates may also act as immune-enhancing agents by activating specialized cancer-killing *gamma-delta T cells* (so-called "gamma-delta therapy"), according to an Italian study published in 2009.[46] In this study, patients with advanced prostate cancer received injections of zoledronate in combination with interleukin-2, an immunotherapy drug. Ninety percent of the patients treated this way either stabilized or improved.[47] Additional trials to evaluate the usefulness of bisphosphonate drugs for cancer treatment are underway.

In general, bisphosphonates are well tolerated by patients and do not produce major side effects. However, use has been associated with *osteonecrosis* of the jaw, a severe bone disease caused by an inadequate blood supply in the area. Although this risk is relatively small, patients should discuss the use of bisphosphonates with their physician prior to beginning a regimen.[48] Their use should be guided and supervised by a healthcare professional.

CALCIUM CHANNEL BLOCKERS

True to their name, calcium channel blockers, also called calcium antagonists, disrupt the movement of calcium through the calcium channels of cells in order to reduce the pressure in the arteries, dilate blood vessels, and relax the heart muscle. This class of drugs is commonly used to treat hypertension (high blood pressure), lessen angina (chest pain), and slow the heart rate.

A calcium channel blocker that may be effective against cancer when combined with chemotherapy is verapamil (Calan, Covera), a drug approved to treat high blood pressure and heart arrhythmias. As discussed in Chapter 1, the effectiveness of certain chemotherapies may be inhibited because of drug-resistant cancer cells that are able to dodge anti-cancer drugs directed at them. Verapamil has been shown to reverse this ability in human cancer cells, thereby increasing the cells' sensitivity to chemotherapy.

Although verapamil's usefulness in cancer treatment has not been confirmed, a number of clinical studies have reported positive results. A French study, for example, used a combination treatment of chemotherapy and verapamil for breast cancer, which produced a higher response rate than chemotherapy treatment alone. Survival also improved by 50 percent.[49] In addition, Japanese scientists found that adding verapamil to standard cancer treatment reduced the recurrence of early-stage bladder cancer.[50]

Calcium channel blockers, including verapamil, can cause serious side effects such as low blood pressure and heart attack. Thus, this class of drugs should be prescribed and closely monitored by the treating physician.

CHELATING AGENTS

Chelating agents, or chelators, are chemical substances designed to remove metallic compounds from the body. Used mainly for treating metal overload or toxicity, this group of agents was first introduced to medicine as an antidote to poison gases during World War I. They were also used widely after World War II, when a large number of navy personnel developed lead poisoning as a result of painting the hulls of ships. Chelating agents were used to remove the lead from their systems.

The scientific rationale for using chelating agents against cancer has to do with the established roles of iron and copper in cancer biology.[51] Iron plays a fundamental part in cell growth, while copper affects angiogenesis. Research has indicated that desferrioxamine (Desferal), a chelator used to treat iron overload, may have potential as a cancer treatment, and iron chelators are currently being developed for this purpose.[52] Likewise, chelating agents like pencillamine (Cuprimine) and trientine (Syprine), which were originally designed to treat disorders caused by copper overload, are now emerging as potential anti-cancer drugs. Tetrathiomolybdate, another pharmaceutical that reduces copper toxicity, is also being studied specifically for the purpose of cancer treatment.[53] The amount of research being done on chelating agents suggests that they may represent a new class of cancer treatment in the future.

Chelators are prescription-only drugs that carry the risk of serious side effects, including anemia and blood clots. They should be taken only as directed by a qualified healthcare professional who will oversee their use.

NARCOTICS

In medicine, the word *narcotic* originally referred to any psychoactive compound that had sleep-inducing properties. Today, the narcotic is generally associated with *opioids*—particularly morphine, heroin, and derivatives such as hydrocodone and codeine—and narcotics themselves are used primarily as painkillers. On occasion, they are used to treat coughs, abdominal cramps, and diarrhea as well. Narcotics also refer to a class of illicit drugs that may be abused. As such, weak narcotics such as methadone (Dolophine, Methadose) are given to recovering addicts to help their bodies detoxify after they stop using dangerous narcotics like heroin.

A weak narcotic that has been increasingly used as an off-label treatment for cancer is naltrexone (Depade, ReVia), a drug normally prescribed to manage alcohol and opioid dependency. So-called *low-dose naltrexone* (LDN) at one-tenth of the dose used for drug rehabilitation has been proposed as a treatment for a broad range of immune disorders. Due to its low toxicity and cost, LDN is becoming a popular off-label cancer treatment as well. Dr. Ian Zagon of Penn State University and the late Dr. Bernard Bihari, an addiction specialist, have been the major driving forces behind the research and popularity of LDN for cancer and other conditions. Dr. Zagon, who has researched opioids and cancer for years, proposed the idea that LDN works in part by interacting with naturally occurring opiates in the body, such as endorphins and opiate receptors, to stimulate the immune system and suppress tumor growth. In the medical literature, there are reported cases of pancreatic cancer successfully treated with LDN and alpha-lipoic acid.[54] There was also a case of lymphoma treated with LDN alone, which caused a reversal of the disease.[55] Clinical trials of LDN are currently in progress to explore its effects on inflammatory bowel disease, multiple sclerosis, and other autoimmune conditions. Similar trials are needed to assess the treatment's effectiveness for cancer.

LDN is not associated with any major side effects, but it should not be taken by patients on narcotic pain medications. Naltrexone should be used with caution by those who have thyroid problems or have had an organ transplant. Patients should follow the directions of their prescribing health practitioner.

STATINS

Statin is the nickname for *HMG-CoA reductase inhibitors*. These drugs are used mainly to treat hyperlipidemia, which is better known as high cholesterol. Statin research was initiated by Japanese scientists in 1971, and the first statin drug—lovastatin (Mevacor)—was developed soon thereafter. Today, statins are one of the most commonly prescribed classes of drugs in the United States, second only to analgesics, and are used to reduce strokes, heart attacks, and levels of cholesterol.

In terms of off-label treatment, statin drugs are particularly interesting because their biological activity is *pleiotropic,* which means they have many other mechanisms besides lowering cholesterol. Scientists are currently researching the usefulness of statins for autoimmune disorders, cataracts, dementia, emphysema, osteoporosis, sepsis, and various cardiovascular conditions. They have also found that statins affect inflammation, immune response, and cell signaling,[56] which suggests that they may have anti-cancer properties, including anti-proliferative, anti-angiogenic, and apoptotic effects.[57] This cancer-fighting potential has been investigated for popular statin drugs like lovastatin, simvastatin (Zocor), atorvastatin (Lipitor), and pravastatin (Pravachol).

Although perhaps not widely known, there is a substantial body of laboratory- and animal-based evidence of the preventative and therapeutic potential of statin drugs for brain, breast, colon, lung, pancreatic, and prostate cancer, among other types. Statins may also have synergistic potential when applied in combination with other anti-cancer agents, especially chemotherapy (doxorubicin, docetaxel, and gemcitabine in particular), radiation, and targeted therapies such as sorafenib (Nexavar). Synergy between statin drugs and unconventional cancer treatments (vitamins, green tea polyphenols, and off-label drugs such as bisphosphonates and COX-2 inhibitors) has also been reported.

There is also clinical data indicating that statin drugs may be effective against cancer in humans. Statins have been shown to reduce cancer incidence and recurrence by as much as 90 percent in colon,[58] breast,[59] lung,[60] liver,[61] and prostate[62] cancer in studies involving nearly half a million patients. People who took statins in high doses or for extended periods of time seemed to benefit the most. According to a study conducted by Japanese researchers, daily doses (40 milligrams) of pravastatin were found to double the survival time of liver cancer patients when used as an adjunctive treatment.[63] Also compelling is the fact that statin drugs can be used in cocktail treatment for both primary and secondary cancer prevention, i.e. preventing cancer occurrence as well as recurrence, especially for breast, colon, lung, and prostate cancer.

Statin drugs are generally very safe; only 3 percent of patients stop taking them due to adverse effects. Common side effects include headaches, muscle aches, and gastrointestinal discomfort. Based on the large volume of research, the benefits of statin use appear to outweigh the potential risks. Still, patients should discuss statin use with a healthcare professional and take the drug only as directed.

THYMIC HORMONES

Thymic hormones are members of the *thymosin family*, which are biologically active molecules produced by the thymus gland. First described by Drs. Goldstein and White in 1966, the immunorestorative effects of thymosins laid the foundation for the first clinical trials of the substance in 1974. These trials found that thymosins "turn on" the immune system in children with *thymic dysplasia*, a rare hereditary condition in which proper function of the thymus gland is impaired, leading to weakened immunity. Today, the role of thymic hormones in immune enhancement has been confirmed in both test-tube and animal studies.[64] Certain thymic fractions, such as thymosin alpha-1 (Zadaxin), are approved drugs in many countries and used to treat immunodeficiency, bone marrow failure, hepatitis B and C, and viral and bacterial infections.[65] Now, the potential use of thymosin alpha-1 as a cancer treatment is also being explored.

Most of the clinical research on oral and injectable thymus extract (see page 128) has been done in Europe, and encouraging results have been reported. Trials have found that cancer patients who are given thymosin alpha-1 while undergoing chemotherapy experience less adverse side effects from the treatment.[66] A large controlled trial in Italy showed close to a 50-percent increase in the survival rate among metastatic melanoma patients treated with thymosin alpha-1 in addition to chemotherapy and immunotherapy.[67] A separate randomized study of liver cancer patients receiving standard treatment along with thymosin alpha-1 also found that survival and tumor response improved.[68] Furthermore, a study of thymosin alpha-1 used in combination with vaccine therapy for breast cancer showed improved response rates by 50 percent.[69] Thymosin alpha-1 is currently undergoing clinical trials in the United States and pending FDA approval.

Since thymic hormones are not yet approved in the United States, patients may substitute with thymus extracts, which are categorized as supplements and do not require prescriptions. However, people with autoimmune disorders should not use thymic peptides unless they are prescribed by a qualified healthcare professional who will closely supervise their use. Thymic hormones should be taken only as directed.

See also Thymus extract.

Dietary Supplements

This section contains a list of vitamins, herbs, and other dietary supplements that may be useful for treating and/or preventing cancer. It is estimated that there are at least 30,000 different dietary supplements in the United States alone, which has a multibillion-dollar market annually and where one in four people take supplements for health enhancement.[1] Unlike drugs, there are no legal provisions requiring the Food and Drug Administration to "approve" dietary supplements based on their safety or effectiveness before they reach the consumer. Nor are there dosage guidelines for dietary supplements of any kind. Moreover, there are only very basic manufacturing standards and regulations in place for many of these compounds, which are not formally inspected for manufacturing consistency. This means that the source and quality of ingredients may vary from product to product; there is no guarantee that the ingredients listed on the products' labels are actually present in their specified amounts, if present at all. Also unlike drugs, most supplements have not undergone extensive research or vigorous clinical trials, and thus carry the disclaimer, "This product is not intended to diagnose, treat, cure, or prevent any disease." Such claims can be made only for pharmaceutical drugs. Due to these limitations, information on the adverse side effects and interactions provided in the following pages should be considered incomplete. It is also important to mention that all specified dosages are recommendations and intended for adults only. Ideally, supplement use should be tailored to the individual taking them—especially in the case of children, as well as women who are pregnant or breastfeeding—and prescribed by a knowledgeable healthcare professional. If you decide to take a supplement, tell your treating physician.

In general, you should always choose products from a reputable manufacturer or distributor, rather than base your choice on price. Additionally, products that contain a single ingredient or only a few are preferable to ones that list a dozen or more ingredients on the label. If you are not sure whether to use a particular supplement, it is wise not to use it. And if you do not understand something written on a supplement label, you should consult your health practitioner or pharmacist before taking the substance. An easy way to learn and compare the ingredients in different products is to visit the Dietary Supplements Labels Database, which is available through the National Library of Medicine website (http://www.nlm.nih.gov/).

The supplements included in the following list can be divided into two basic categories. First, there are supplements that have recently undergone independent clinical studies in humans and have demonstrated effectiveness against cancer. Also included are supplements that are commonly used by cancer patients, but are not adequately supported by science. These substances, which are identified by an asterisk (*) next to their names, are not necessarily endorsed by this book.

ASTRAGALUS

Astragalus is an herb used in Traditional Chinese Medicine, as well as by herbalists and alternative health practitioners in the West, primarily to enhance the body's *qi,* or energy. The biologically active ingredients of astragalus include polysaccharides, beta-sitosterol, saponins, and flavonoids.[2] Astragalus stimulates the growth of bone marrow stem cells, promotes the maturation of stem cells into white blood cells, and activates white blood cells—specifically, macrophages, T-cells, and natural killer (NK) cells—to enhance the immune system. In China, astragalus root is often used as an adjuvant to chemotherapy, either alone or as an ingredient in an herbal formula. A review of thirty-four randomized studies—which involved 2,815 patients who received astragalus-based Chinese herbal formulas in combination with platinum-based chemotherapy—found that thirty of these studies showed improvement in patient response to treatment. Twelve studies showed improvement in survival.[3]

In Traditional Chinese Medicine, the astragalus root is usually used in soups and teas, or taken as an extract or as a capsule. Although there are many grades and forms of the herb, the general dosage ranges from 9 to 15 grams daily or the equivalent amount of the dry herb, which may be taken in the form of a tea decoction, a concentrated extract, or a capsule. Astragalus has not been known to cause clinical toxicity, but patients should consult a knowledgeable healthcare professional before taking the herb and should use astragalus only as directed.

CAROTENOIDS

See Lycopene; Vitamin A.

CARTILAGE, SHARK* AND BOVINE

The interest in using shark cartilage as a cancer treatment began around the same time that Dr. Judah Folkman discovered that angiogenesis was a growth mechanism for cancer, thus making anti-angiogenesis a goal of treatment. A 1983 article in the journal *Science* described shark cartilage as containing a substance that inhibits the growth of blood vessels, which, in turn, restricts tumor growth. But it was a 1993 episode of *60 Minutes* that called attention to the role of angiogenesis in cancer growth and popularized the idea that "sharks don't get cancer." This led to the widespread—and controversial— use of shark cartilage as an alternative cancer treatment. But even as angiogenesis became established medical knowledge, key trials using shark cartilage to treat cancer yielded negative results,[4] and its use has since dramatically diminished.

Bovine cartilage, though never as popular as shark cartilage, is actually better validated by science. Nearly two decades before shark cartilage became widely touted as a cancer treatment, Dr. John F. Prudden, originally of Columbia Presbyterian Medical Center in New York, began to study the effects of cartilage on cancer. He reported that a number of his cancer patients significantly responded to bovine cartilage extract.[5] At the same time, a phase II trial of the extract reported a complete remission in one metastatic kidney cancer patient.[6] Subsequently, a team from New York Medical College conducted a separate clinical trial testing the effects of bovine cartilage on metastatic kidney cancer. Of the twenty-two patients who participated in the trial, three patients had objective, measurable responses to the treatment. None of the patients had relapsed as of their six-month, twelve-month, and thirty-month follow-ups.[7]

The usual dose of bovine cartilage is 3 grams taken orally three times a day. There have not been any significant side effects reported, but patients should speak to a healthcare professional before taking this supplement, and use it only as directed.

COENZYME Q_{10}*

Coenzyme Q_{10}—also known as ubiquinone, CoQ_{10}, or Q_{10}—is a widely available and commonly used supplement. It is naturally found in cells and is involved in a number of cellular processes, in addition to acting as an antioxidant in the body. CoQ_{10} supplements are used to prevent cardiovascular conditions, especially heart failure, as well as periodontal disease and muscular dystrophy. The supplement may also boost energy and speed recovery from exercise. Its role in cancer treatment originated in 1961, when scientists discovered that the blood of cancer patients contained little coenzyme Q_{10}. Subsequently, other researchers suggested that CoQ_{10} may help the immune system and, therefore, could be used as a cancer treatment.

Although there have not been controlled trials of coenzyme Q_{10} for cancer treatment, a handful of patients have provided anecdotal accounts of its benefits. In addition, the biochemist Dr. Karl Folkers reported that the cancer of many patients who used CoQ_{10} went into remission.[8] Specifically, there were reported benefits for patients with breast and prostate cancer who took CoQ_{10} in doses of up to 600 milligrams per day. (This study was never published due in large part to Dr. Folkers' death.) It was later reported that some cancer patients who followed a nutritional program including coenzyme Q_{10} experienced tumor shrinkage, though it is not clear if this can be specifically attributed to the supplement.[9] A more scientifically valid application of CoQ_{10} in the treatment of cancer is reducing the *cardiotoxicity*, or heart muscle damage, caused by certain chemotherapy drugs.[10]

Based on Dr. Folkers' research, the recommended daily dose of coenzyme Q_{10} for cancer is 300 milligrams or more. The supplement is generally safe, but taking 100 milligrams or more per day may cause mild insomnia in some people. Additionally, some research has detected elevated levels of liver enzymes in those taking 300 milligrams per day for long periods of time. CoQ_{10} may also interact with blood thinners such as warfarin (Coumadin), so daily use of the supplement should always be monitored by a qualified healthcare professional.

CURCUMIN

Curcumin is a complex compound that has been used medicinally for thousands of years. It is the principal bioactive ingredient of *turmeric,* a popular Indian spice used in foods such as curry. Because it has multiple biological targets and cellular effects, curcumin has been used to treat a wide spectrum of ailments, including cancer. The compound has anti-tumor potential due to its anti-inflammatory and immunomodulatory properties, as well as its ability to inhibit cancer invasion, angiogenesis, and metastasis.[11] The laboratory evidence of curcumin's effectiveness against cancer is so impressive that Dr. Razelle Kurzrock, the department chairperson of MD Anderson Cancer Center's Investigational Cancer Therapeutics Program, has said, "It was clear that this agent was just as potent at killing tumor cells in the lab as any experimental drug I'd seen from pharmaceutical companies."

However, one concern about curcumin is its poor absorption upon being ingested. There is also relatively limited data confirming its cancer-fighting effectiveness in humans, though it has been preliminarily tested in combination with the chemotherapy drugs 5-fluorouracil, oxaliplatin, gemcitabine, and taxanes for the treatment of gastrointestinal, breast, and prostate cancers. A recent French trial of paclitaxel (Taxol) chemotherapy combined with curcumin for advanced breast cancer yielded encouraging results, and a trial that was conducted at the MD Anderson Cancer Center demonstrated similarly promising results among a small number of pancreatic cancer patients.[12]

Curcumin has not been known to cause any significant toxicity—a trial using up to 8,000 milligrams of curcumin per day for three months in humans found no toxic effects. Still, curcumin is a spice, so it may cause mild gastrointestinal side effects like nausea and diarrhea when consumed in large quantities. The recommended dosage ranges from 3,600 to 8,000 milligrams a day. The correct dosage should be prescribed by the healthcare professional who will oversee its use.

D-GLUCARIC ACID

Also known as D-glucarate and calcium D-glucarate, D-glucaric acid is a nontoxic compound contained in many vegetables and fruits, with the highest concentrations found in apples, grapefruit, oranges, and cruciferous vegetables. The body also naturally produces the compound in small amounts.

D-glucaric acid and its derivatives exert anti-cancer action in part by changing the body's hormonal environment, which is why they may be particularly useful for hormone-dependent cancers, such as breast and prostate cancer. D-glucarates also suppress cell proliferation and inflammation, induce apoptosis, and activate detoxification pathways in the body, which allows for the removal of foreign toxins and excess hormones. D-glucarate supplements can help to boost the body's natural defense mechanism for eliminating harmful carcinogens and other cancer-causing agents.[13] In laboratory testing, D-glucaric acid has been shown to have a modest preventive effect for various tumors, and an anti-proliferative effect on estrogen-sensitive breast tumor cells.[14]

Toxic side effects have not been reported for D-glucaric acid. When taken in the form of calcium D-glucarate supplements, the usual suggested dose is 1,500 milligrams (containing 180 milligrams of calcium) three times per day with meals. Although there are no known side effects, patients should consult a healthcare professional before supplementing with D-glucarates and use these substances only as directed.

DHA

See Omega-3 fatty acids.

DIINDOLYLMETHANE (DIM)

The anti-cancer properties of bioactive substances found in cruciferous vegetables like broccoli, Brussels sprouts, cauliflower, and cabbage have been increasingly recognized. Among the substances derived from such foods is *3,3'-diindolylmethane,* or DIM, which is produced in the acidic environment of the stomach following the ingestion of vegetables containing indole-3-carbinol. (To learn more about indole-3-carbinol, see page 119.) Researchers have explored the ability of DIM to prevent, inhibit, and reverse the progression of cancer, and clinical trials are underway to test its use in treating the disease.[15]

Studies have shown that DIM can affect cancer cells in diverse ways. One pilot placebo-controlled study used DIM to treat *cervical dysplasia,* a precancerous condition indicated by abnormal pap smears. Sixty-four female patients with this condition took 2 milligrams of DIM per kilogram of their body weight (mg/kg) every day for three months. Following treatment, the pap smears of nearly half of the patients either normalized or improved, with no significant toxic effects.[16]

The usual suggested dose of DIM is 150 to 300 milligrams per day, and it should be taken with a light meal to enhance its absorption. While there are no known serious side effects, patients should consult a healthcare professional before supplementing with DIM and use the substance only as directed.

EGCG

See Green tea.

EPA

See Omega-3 fatty acids.

ESSIAC TEA*

The word *Essiac* is the reverse spelling of "Caisse," the last name of the Canadian nurse who first promoted the use of this herbal tea mixture in the 1920s. It is rumored that a Native American medicine man from the Ojibwa tribe gave the mixture to a cancer patient, who, in turn, gave it to Rene Caisse. Essiac is based on four herbs—burdock root, Indian rhubarb root, sheep sorrel, and slippery elm bark—but others may be included depending on the manufacturer. It has been claimed that Essiac removes toxins from the body, strengthens the immune system, reduces tumor size, increases cancer survival, and improves overall quality of life. Today, it is among the most popular supplements for cancer.

Despite this popularity, however, there have not been any trials testing Essiac or similar formulas (for example, Flor-Essence) for cancer. The most information we have about Essiac's potential usefulness is based on a series of cases in Canada. In the 1980s, the Canadian Department of National Health and Welfare reviewed eighty-six cancer cases submitted by physicians who had given Essiac to their patients. The review found that forty-seven patients did not benefit from the tea; eight patients objectively improved or remained stable; five patients required less pain medication; one patient felt physically better but did not actually improve; and the remaining patients could not be evaluated. Following further investigation, however, researchers discovered that of the eight patients who were reported as being stable, three had worsened and two patients had died. Moreover, the remaining three patients who actually stabilized after using Essiac tea had received conventional treatments as well, so their improvement could not be definitively attributed to Essiac.[17]

Operating out of Massachusetts General Hospital, the Natural Standard Research Collaboration reviewed Essiac in 2009 and concluded that the tea had not sufficiently demonstrated efficacy against cancer.[18] As such, Essiac is an example of a popular anti-cancer remedy that lacks adequate scientific evidence to support its use.

FISH OIL

See Omega-3 fatty acids.

GAMMA-LINOLENIC ACID (GLA)

Gamma-linolenic acid, or GLA, is an anti-inflammatory bioactive fatty acid usually extracted from borage or evening primrose oil. Numerous test-tube studies have confirmed the ability of GLA to induce apoptosis (cancer cell death), promote anti-angiogenesis, favorably alter gene expression, and enhance the potency of chemotherapy and radiation therapy.[19] Laboratory studies have shown that more than forty different human cancer types can be killed by GLA, and some researchers have proposed GLA as a new nontoxic cancer therapy. Another significant anti-cancer action of GLA is its ability to affect cells' hormone receptors, and researchers have investigated the effects of GLA on hormone-sensitive cancers such as breast and prostate cancer. In one study, breast cancer patients took eight capsules of GLA (a total of 2.8 grams) per day while receiving standard hormone therapy. This combination treatment produced better responses than hormone therapy after only six weeks.[20] In another study, directly applying GLA to brain tumors or nearby tissues during surgery resulted in cancer regressions and improvements in survival among brain cancer patients.[21]

Yet, GLA may not be safe for everyone. There have been reports of seizures in people taking evening primrose oil, a substance from which GLA is derived. As such, people taking phenothiazines, a class of medications used to treat psychosis, should avoid taking GLA because the combination may increase the risk of seizures. Those planning to have surgery requiring anesthesia should stop taking GLA two weeks prior to the procedure, since it may interact with anesthesia medications. In addition, because the substance may increase the risk of bleeding, patients on blood thinners should avoid supplements containing GLA.

The usual dosage of GLA is 480 to 3,000 milligrams taken over the course of the day. The actual dose depends on the condition being treated and should be prescribed by a healthcare professional who will oversee its use.

GENISTEIN

See Soy isoflavones.

GLUTAMINE

Also known as L-glutamine, glutamine is normally a nonessential amino acid and the most plentiful protein building block in the body. In times of bodily stress, however, this amino acid may become conditionally essential in order to maintain the healthy function of tissues. Glutamine protects the cells and tissues, reduces inflammation, and helps maintain proper metabolic function, among several other important mechanisms. Current evidence supports the use of glutamine for *sepsis*—a dangerous condition in which the bloodstream becomes infected with bacteria—as well as severe burns among the intensive-care population.

Glutamine was nicknamed "the indispensable nutrient in oncology" by researchers who found that the amino acid is beneficial for cancer patients, a discovery based on a review of thirty-six clinical studies published on the topic within the past two decades.[22] Specifically, glutamine may decrease the incidence and severity of chemotherapy-associated diarrhea, neuropathy, heart damage, and *mucositis*—inflammation of the digestive tract.[23] In addition to reducing the toxicity of chemotherapy and radiation, experimental data indicates that glutamine diminishes tumor growth by improving metabolism, thereby restoring the function of specific immune cells, such as natural killer (NK) cells.

People with kidney or liver dysfunction should not supplement with glutamine without approval from their physician. The normal dosage range is 15 to 30 grams daily, divided into three 5- to 10-gram doses taken over the course of the day. Most often, glutamine supplements are taken in the form of a powder blended with a liquid. The use of glutamine by cancer patients receiving chemotherapy and radiation treatment should be monitored by a qualified and experienced healthcare professional.

GREEN TEA

Tea made from the *Camellia sinensis* plant is one of the most studied and consumed beverages worldwide due to its reported health benefits. In recent years, epidemiological, laboratory, animal, and human studies have all found that the bioactive compounds in tea may help prevent cancer.[24] Laboratory studies show that some components of green tea can cause cancer cells to stop dividing in a phenomenon known as *cell arrest,* as well as induce apoptosis, or cell death. Moreover, animal studies have shown that green tea inhibits tumor growth in various organ sites, including the skin, lungs, liver, stomach, breast, and colon.

The tea plant, especially unfermented green tea, is particularly rich in compounds known as *catechins,* which are thought to be the major anti-cancer component. The main active catechin is a substance known as *epigallocatechin 3-gallate,* or EGCG. This substance, which has been the major focus of research on tea's anti-cancer effects, works against the disease by influencing cell growth via the regulation of multiple cellular signal pathways.[25] One 6-ounce cup (about 173 grams) of brewed green tea has approximately 235 milligrams of catechins—about 45 milligrams of EGCG.[26] However, the actual EGCG content can be quite varied depending on the type and age of the tea, as well as how the tea is prepared. Most of the research pointing to the health benefits of green tea is based on its consumption among Asian populations, since the average individual consumes between 60 to 100 milligrams of EGCG per day. For cancer prevention and treatment, studies have used green tea extracts containing 300 milligrams to 2 grams of EGCG daily, which is the equivalent of anywhere from seven to twenty 6-ounce cups of brewed green tea.

There is also population-based evidence of green tea's effectiveness for ovarian and prostate cancer prevention. Larsson and Wolk from the famed Karolinska Institute in Sweden analyzed the relationship between tea intake and ovarian cancer rates in a study involving 61,057 women, and found a lower risk of ovarian cancer among tea drinkers. Women who drank one cup per day lowered their risk by 24 percent, and those who drank two or more cups a day reduced their risk by 46 percent.[27] Another study found that women with ovarian cancer who drank at least one cup of green tea daily lowered their risk of death by 56 percent over the course of the three-year study.[28] For breast cancer, a Harvard review of studies conducted between 1998 and 2009 identified a relationship between drinking green tea (at least three cups per day) and reduced recurrence of the disease.[29]

Furthermore, a large Japanese study involving almost 50,000 men found that drinking tea was correlated with reduced incidence of advanced prostate cancer.[30] Also notable is a recent cancer prevention study of the effects of green tea supplements (200-milligram doses taken three times a day) in men. Of the thirty men who took the supplements, only one was diagnosed with prostate cancer after one year. In comparison, there were nine diagnoses among the thirty men given a placebo.[31] Researchers at MD Anderson Cancer Center have also noted that green tea extract has a positive effect on people with a precancerous condition called oral leukoplakia. More than half of patients who took the extract were less likely to develop cancer than those who did not.[32]

Studies employing green tea as an actual cancer treatment (and not just as a preventative) are fewer in number but encouraging nonetheless. After four leukemia patients reportedly responded to green tea treatment alone,[33] the Mayo Clinic conducted a trial in which early-stage chronic lymphocytic leukemia patients were given .4 to 2 grams of EGCG daily. The results were positive, showing clinical improvement in a majority of patients.[34] In yet another study, 800 milligrams of EGCG in a mixture totaling 1.3 grams of tea polyphenols were given to prostate cancer patients scheduled to undergo prostatectomies. After receiving this treatment for only a short time, blood tests showed significant reductions in their prostate-specific antigen (PSA) levels, a biomarker for prostate cancer.[35]

Brewed green tea and green tea extract are generally safe and lacking in side effects. Still, it is important to remember that tea contains caffeine, which may cause mild to moderate side effects, including insomnia and nervousness in those who are sensitive to the substance. According to a phase I trial at Memorial Sloan-Kettering Cancer Center, the maximum dose of brewed green tea that people can tolerate is approximately 2.5 liters (or about 2.1 quarts) per day.[36]

It is also possible that some drugs may negatively interact with catechins and EGCG. In particular, the cancer drug bortezomib (Velcade), which is used to treat myeloma and certain lymphomas, can be neutralized by EGCG. Therefore, cancer patients receiving this treatment should not drink or supplement with green tea. Green tea supplements for cancer treatment should be prescribed and monitored by an experienced health practitioner.

HERBS, CHINESE

See Traditional Chinese Medicine.

INDOLE-3-CARBINOL (I3C)

Indole-3-carbinol (I3C) is produced by the cruciferous family of vegetables, which includes broccoli, Brussels sprouts, cabbage, cauliflower, daikon, and radishes. In the body, I3C is converted to a series of end products, such as DIM (see page 113), that may alter hormone metabolism, particularly the female sex hormone estrogen. This suggests that I3C may be useful primarily for hormonally driven cancers, and test-tube experiments have demonstrated that I3C suppresses the proliferation of tumor cells in breast, prostate, endometrial, and colon cancer.[37] Human-based studies on early-stage gynecological cancers have found that the substance can alleviate cancer-related symptoms, as well as improve disease pathology.[38] Furthermore, I3C may be beneficial for preventing breast cancer.

Although there are no significant side effects associated with I3C use, researchers have expressed concern about the chemical instability of I3C—it rapidly converts to other molecules upon reaching the stomach. In addition, some medical scientists believe that much of I3C's biological activity is really carried out by DIM, one of its byproducts. Controversies aside, the smallest dose that is believed to have an anti-cancer effect is 300 milligrams per day.[39] Use of I3C should be guided by an experienced health professional, and patients should take the substance only as directed.

INOSITOL HEXAPHOSPHATE (IP-6)

Inositol hexaphosphate, also known as IP-6 and phytic acid, is a naturally occurring carbohydrate present in many plant sources, as well as certain high-fiber foods like rice bran cereal and legumes. The majority of research on IP-6, which has been shown to regulate vital cell functions such as growth, has been conducted by Abulkalam Shamsuddin, a scientist at the University of Maryland's School of Medicine. In cases of leukemia and breast, colon, liver, prostate, and skin cancer, IP-6 has been shown to prevent angiogenesis and enhance the immune system.[40]

IP-6 is safe and does not produce any significant side effects when taken in normal doses—which is why a recent review states that there is "clearly enough evidence to justify the initiation of Phase I and Phase II clinical trials (of IP-6) in humans."[41] Indeed, an issue with IP-6 is the relative lack of clinical studies, though there is preliminary animal-based data showing that it may prevent cancer, and clinical data indicating that the substance may control cancer's spread and improve quality of life.[42]

IP-6 may reduce platelet activity and, therefore, should be carefully administered to people who have low blood cell counts or take blood thinning medication. Since it is an antioxidant, IP-6 may not be appropriate treatment for patients receiving radiation or certain chemotherapies, which kill cancer cells partly by way of oxidation. The usual recommended dose for the purpose of cancer prevention is 1 to 2 grams daily on an empty stomach, 4 grams daily for people with an increased risk of cancer, and up to 8 grams daily for those who already have been diagnosed. Dosage amounts should be prescribed and monitored by a qualified healthcare professional who will oversee the use of the supplement.

LYCOPENE

Lycopene is a bright red pigment found in fruits and vegetables such as tomatoes, watermelons, and papayas. Population-based studies have found an inverse relationship between tomato consumption and cancer risk, which is why lycopene is considered a potential preventative for cancer, especially prostate cancer. The anti-cancer properties of lycopene are well established, as the substance has been found to inhibit breast, endometrial, prostate, and colon cancer cells. Consuming lycopene has also been associated with fewer cancer-related symptoms overall. [43]

The majority of research on lycopene's anti-cancer potential has focused specifically on prostate cancer. Not only may the substance prevent the disease, but it may also lower PSA levels in prostate cancer patients, according to a recent review of related studies. In a small study involving twenty prostate cancer patients treated with lycopene, the disease progressed in only 15 percent of patients, while 35 percent of patients significantly responded to the treatment. [44]

Lycopene does not have any known significant side effects. The daily recommended dosage is 10 to 15 milligrams, but patients should consult a healthcare professional to determine a dose appropriate for their individual needs. The supplement should be taken only as directed by the treating health practitioner.

MELATONIN

A naturally occurring antioxidant, melatonin is normally produced and secreted by the pineal gland to regulate the sleep-wake cycle. In addition to its primary biological functions, melatonin may be beneficial for a variety of health conditions, including sleep problems, immune disorders, and cancer. Although it is regulated as a drug in many parts of the world, melatonin is considered a supplement in the United States.

Melatonin stands out as a dietary supplement because its effectiveness as a cancer treatment has been confirmed by clinical trials. Studies have shown that melatonin can inhibit various cancers via multiple mechanisms, including anti-angiogensis, immune enhancement, and apoptosis. Notably, ten randomized controlled trials—which were conducted by Dr. Paoli Lissoni's team from 1992 to 2003 and involved 643 cancer patients—discovered that survival significantly improved when treatment programs included melatonin.[45] Another trial of melatonin supplements combined with conventional treatments for liver cancer resulted in fewer treatment-related side effects, and improved the two-year survival rate among participating patients by 50 percent.[46] Treatment regimens including melatonin also caused some cancers to regress and prolonged the survival of patients with other types of cancer, including leukemia. Furthermore, there is evidence that melatonin may reduce chemotherapy-induced neuropathy, as well as low lymphocyte white blood cell counts caused by radiation.[47]

Based upon the studies done by Dr. Lissoni's group, melatonin may be effective in doses of 20 to 40 milligrams per day. The supplement should be taken in the evening, since it is likely to cause drowsiness. Melatonin may also cause headaches, nausea, nightmares, irritability, dizziness, and depression. The use of this agent for cancer treatment and/or prevention should be prescribed and closely monitored by a qualified healthcare professional.

MODIFIED CITRUS PECTIN

Modified citrus pectin is a complex polysaccharide extracted from the peel and pulp of citrus fruits, and is typically used to remove heavy metals from the body.[48] There is not an abundance of cancer-related research on this substance, but scientists have so far determined that it can prevent cancer metastasis.[49] Most of the published studies on the use of modified citrus pectin for cancer have used animals, not humans, as subjects, and have focused on breast, colon, and prostate cancer. One small pilot study found that it may slow the growth of prostate cancer.

Modified citrus pectin, available in either capsule or powder form, is generally safe. The dose suggested by manufacturers is 5 grams (about one-fifth of an ounce) for the powder, which is mixed with water or juice and taken three times per day with meals. For capsules, the suggested dose is 800 milligrams, which should also be taken with meals three times per day.

OMEGA-3 FATTY ACIDS

Omega-3 fatty acids, such as *docosahexaenoic acid* (DHA) and *eicosapentaenoic acid* (EPA), are essential fatty acids required for human health. Their healing effect on various diseases from cardiovascular conditions to psychological disorders has long been studied. The biological activities of omega-3 fatty acids specific to cancer include reducing inflammation, slowing tumor growth and angiogenesis, and inducing apoptosis. In addition, omega-3 supplements, which may enhance chemotherapy and radiation,[50] have been found to work synergistically with COX-2 inhibitors, genistein, and other anti-cancer compounds. However, there have not been any trials involving human patients to verify these potential effects, and the cancer-fighting properties of omega-3s in humans have not yet been confirmed.

Although there is no clear evidence that omega-3 fatty acids can treat or prevent cancer, they may improve the life quality of cancer patients. More specifically, omega-3s seem to effectively combat *cachexia,* a condition that frequently occurs among advanced-stage cancer patients that results in loss of appetite and significant weight reduction. A review of seventeen related studies revealed that administering EPA and DHA to advanced cancer patients in daily doses of at least 1.5 grams for a prolonged period of time improved life quality.[51] So, even though it is not clear if omega-3s can actually block the growth of cancer or improve survival, there is preliminary evidence that they enhance patients' quality of life.

When taken in normal doses, omega-3 fatty acids have not produced significant side effects. However, consuming more than 3 grams per day may increase the risk of bleeding in people who take anticoagulant drugs. A suggested dosage for cancer-related weight or appetite loss is 1,600 milligrams per day, but patients should consult a healthcare professional to determine a dosage appropriate for their needs. The supplement should be used only as directed by a healthcare professional.

PAU D'ARCO*

Also known as Red Lapacho (*Tabebuia impetiginosa*), Pau d'arco is a tree found in the Amazon that has been touted as a cure for a cancer since the 1960s. Traditionally, it is consumed as a tea prepared from the inner bark of the tree and used to treat conditions such as infections, stomach problems, and bladder disorders. The primary bioactive compounds that have been isolated from Pau d'arco are *lapachol* and *beta-lapachone*, which is considered the main anti-tumor compound of the plant. Although Pau d'arco appears to be safe, there are no published clinical studies verifying its effectiveness against cancer. Therefore, despite its popularity, it cannot be recommended.

PSP AND PSK†

Derived from the *Coriolus versicolor* mushroom and related to health-promoting polysaccharides like beta-glucan, PSP and PSK are just two of many mushroom-based nutritional supplements that have been shown to enhance the immune system. PSP and PSK are well established in terms of clinical efficacy, with positive trial data for esophageal, gastric, colorectal, breast, nasopharyngeal, and lung cancer, as well as acute leukemia, both with and without chemotherapy.[52]

There are no known significant side effects or toxicities associated with PSP and PSK. The usual dose for PSK is 3 grams a day, while effective doses of PSP are slightly higher, at 9 grams a day. Use of these supplements should be monitored by a qualified healthcare professional.

---

†Although naturally derived, PSK (Krestin) is a registered pharmaceutical in Japan, and not considered a supplement. Most of the clinical trials related to PSK have been carried out in Japan.

RED YEAST RICE

Also called *monascus,* red yeast rice is a popular supplement consisting of a type of yeast that has been used in Asia as a food preservative and colorant for centuries. One of its many bioactive ingredients is monacolin K, which is identical to lovastatin, the original statin drug. Therefore, when taken in equivalent doses, the effectiveness of red yeast rice as a cancer treatment is comparable to statin drugs (see page 104). Test-tube studies have confirmed these cancer-inhibiting properties.

The side effects of red yeast rice are similar to the effects of statins and include *myopathy,* or muscle inflammation and dysfunction. The usual recommended dose for adults is between 600 and 1,200 milligrams per day, but exact dosage amounts should be tailored to the individual. Patients should take the substance only as directed by a healthcare professional.

RUTA-6

Derived from the *Ruta graveolens* plant, Ruta-6 is a homeopathic medicine that was first advocated as a cancer treatment by Dr. Prasanta Banerji of Calcutta, India, who has pioneered its use. Other homeopathic medicines—such as Hydrastis, Lycopodium, Carcinosin, Phytolacca, Conium, and thuja—have been used as cancer treatments, but Ruta-6 was proven to be a more powerful agent in a study involving mice.[53] The substance may be especially beneficial for treating brain cancer.[54] Although Dr. Banerji claimed that the substance brought about complete remissions for 21 percent of his cancer patients, this percentage seems unusually high.[55] Nevertheless, Ruta-6 supplementation is worth considering for cancer treatment, since it is inexpensive and has not been known to cause side effects.

Generally, dosage amounts should be determined on an individual basis and prescribed by a homeopathic doctor. As a reference, the dosage most often recommended by Dr. Banerji is three homeopathic Ruta-6 pills along with three homeopathic calcium phosphate (3X- or 6X-strength) pills per day. He advises patients to take one Ruta-6 pill at 7:00 AM, 1:00 PM, and 7:00 PM under the tongue, and one calcium phosphate pill at 10:00 AM, 4:00 PM, and 10:00 PM, also under the tongue. As an alternative, patients can take two Ruta-6 pills twice per day—two in the morning and two in the evening—in addition to two calcium phosphate (3X- or 6X-strength) pills per day, one at noon and the other at bedtime. Patients should consult a qualified healthcare professional before using the supplement, and take it only as directed.

SELENIUM

A non-metallic chemical element with industrial applications, selenium first gained attention as a medicinal substance when scientists discovered its ability to protect against liver damage in rats. Since then, there have been more than 200 animal studies evaluating selenium's anti-cancer potential, with positive results reported in more than two-thirds of these studies. Three major studies focused on its use for cancer prevention in humans, and these too had positive results. In particular, a landmark observational study at Cornell University involving 8,629 patient-years showed that 200 micrograms of selenium per day significantly reduced the incidence of lung, colorectal, and prostate cancer.[56] However, selenium has not proven effective for actually treating the disease in humans.

For cancer prevention, selenium should be taken in 200-microgram doses once a day. It is important to keep in mind that the total daily intake of selenium from all sources—food and supplements—should be less than 400 micrograms, which is the largest dose that is considered safe. Excessive selenium intake can cause toxicity, which may be characterized by symptoms such as diarrhea, fatigue, hair loss, joint pain, nausea, and nail discoloration and brittleness.[57] An experienced healthcare professional should be consulted before taking selenium.

SOY ISOFLAVONES

Cultivated for more than 3,000 years, soy is a nutritious plant that can be consumed whole or as soymilk, soy oil, tofu, miso, and tempeh, among other forms. Soy contains bioactive ingredients called *isoflavones*, which are structurally similar to estrogen and, therefore, also known as *phytoestrogens*. The medicinal properties of soy are derived mainly from these isoflavones, particularly *genistein*. Studies have shown that genistein can inhibit the spread of cancer by hindering cell growth via gene modulation. In addition to its anti-metastatic and anti-angiogenic properties, genistein also influences sex hormone signaling in cells, suggesting that it may work against hormonally driven cancers like prostate and breast cancer.

Yet, the use of soy against breast cancer has been controversial and confusing.[58] On the one hand, there are population-based studies showing that soy intake protects against breast cancer.[59] However, because isoflavones can stimulate estrogen-sensitive breast cancer cells, soy may actually promote the growth of the disease. Such adverse effects have been demonstrated in laboratory studies.

In contrast, the benefits of soy for prostate cancer seem more definitive. A review of thirteen studies concluded that consuming soy and soy products can lower the risk of the disease.[60] In addition, a representative Canadian study found that the PSA of prostate cancer patients declined in nearly half of those who drank 500 milliliters of soy-based beverages daily for six months.[61] These results confirmed similar findings of an earlier study conducted in the Netherlands.[62]

To date, there have not been any reported side effects of either short- or long-term use of soy. However, soy isoflavones are known to produce mild estrogen-like side effects. In light of the current controversy, it is advisable for breast cancer patients to avoid soy and soy products, especially if they are undergoing hormone therapy. Studies on soy intake indicate that consuming 25 to 50 grams of soy protein per day (the equivalent of approximately 25 to 50 milligrams of soy isoflavones), has health benefits. For treating prostate cancer, the recommended dose of soy isoflavones is 100 to 120 milligrams per day, which is the amount that has been used in various trials. Consuming soy from dietary sources is generally safe (except in the case of some breast cancer patients), but soy supplements should be taken only under the careful monitoring of a healthcare professional.

THYMUS EXTRACT

Located near the thyroid, the *thymus* is a gland that plays a significant role in regulating immune function. It produces *T-lymphocytes*, a type of white blood cell, as well as various hormones that affect immunity.[63] Thymus extract is usually derived from bovines, and can be found in capsule or tablet form. The substance seems to be safe for most people, but since it typically comes from animals, there have been concerns about disease transmission. So far, though, there have not been any reported cases of disease in humans due to contaminated thymus extract.

Thymic peptide and thymic hormone supplements should be avoided by patients with autoimmune disorders such as systemic lupus erythematosus (SLE), rheumatoid arthritis, and thyroiditis. A typical daily dose is 750 milligrams of crude thymus polypeptide fraction, or 120 milligrams of pure thymus polypeptides (thymomodulin). Thymus supplements should be taken only under the supervision of an experienced and knowledgeable healthcare professional.

See also Thymic hormones.

TOCOTRIENOLS

Tocotrienols are members of the antioxidant vitamin-E family, which consists of four tocopherols and four tocotrienols—alpha, beta, gamma, and delta. Since the vast majority of research on vitamin E pertains to tocopherols, tocotrienols are relatively underappreciated. But evidence shows that tocotrienols are much more potent than the more common tocopherol form of E vitamins, especially against cancer.[64]

Tocotrienols were first discovered by Pennock and Whittle in 1964, but it was not until the 1990s that their anti-cancer properties were first noticed. Both in the laboratory and in animals, tocotrienols have been shown to inhibit cell growth, regulate the cell growth cycle, induce apoptosis, and block angiogenesis. According to a number of studies, tocotrienols may be effective against a host of cancers, including breast, pancreatic, prostate, and skin cancer. Tocotrienols also work synergistically with many substances, including statin drugs like simvastatin (Zocor), COX-2 inhibitors, estrogen-receptor modulators (tamoxifen), green tea polyphenols (EGCG), tyrosine kinase inhibitors like erlotinib (Tarceva), and certain chemotherapies.[65]

TRADITIONAL CHINESE MEDICINE (TCM)

Unlike the other items discussed within these pages, Traditional Chinese Medicine (TCM) is not a treatment agent or even a group of agents. Like homeopathy and Ayurveda, Traditional Chinese Medicine is a distinct system of treatment based on a complex understanding of the body that involves vital energies (qi) and a delicate balance of elements (yin and yang). There are a few well-known TCM remedies, such as acupuncture and green tea, but the system also utilizes a large pharmacopoeia of natural therapies. These therapies are based primarily on herbs and include minerals, marine creatures, and insects. The anti-cancer potential of hundreds of substances commonly used in TCM—astragalus (see page 108) and PSP mushroom extract (see page 124), for example—has been verified by modern science.*

TCM herbal formulas (or "Fu Fang") are based on the principle of cocktail therapy, and the array of potential ingredients is vast. Some of the substances contained in these traditional formulas have been researched in the Western world and developed into cytotoxic cancer drugs. For example, the anti-cancer drug Camptosar (irinotecan), which is used mainly to treat colorectal cancer, was derived and modified from the Chinese tree *Camptotheca acuminata*. Another example is the leukemia drug arsenic trioxide, an indirect derivative of the Chinese herb Indigo naturalis.

Other drugs based on Traditional Chinese Medicine undoubtedly await discovery—many herbs and formulas commonly used in TCM have immunomodulatory[66] and anti-angiogenic[67] mechanisms, among other anti-cancer properties. Clinical trials have found that TCM herbal formulas can prolong survival, reduce side effects of conventional cancer treatments, and improve patients' quality of life when combined with standard therapies.[68] TCM herbs and formulas may be used as adjunctive cancer treatments[69] or as preventative agents.[70]

---

*See Asian Anti-Cancer Database project site at www.asiancancerherb.info for details. The site lists almost 700 potentially anti-cancer materia medica mainly of traditional Chinese origin, including terrestrial plants (80 percent), fungi (9 percent), food (3.5 percent), marine life (1.8 percent), reptiles (1.2 percent), and minerals (1 percent).

While there have been numerous laboratory studies, human-based research on tocotrienols is not as plentiful. Currently, a phase I study evaluating the effects of a pure tocotrienol on pancreatic cancer is underway at the H. Lee Moffitt Cancer Center in Florida.

Gamma and delta tocotrienols, the forms typically used in cancer research, have not been found to cause toxicity in humans. In clinical trials, doses as low as 42 milligrams per day have produced biological effects, but 240 milligrams per day is the recommended dosage for cancer prevention and/or treatment. Based on studies in humans, this amount does not have adverse side effects or toxicities when taken for up to forty-eight months. Even so, patients should consult a healthcare professional before supplementing with tocotrienols.

TURMERIC

See Curcumin.

VITAMIN A

"Vitamin A" is a broad term that encompasses a large number of related compounds that have diverse roles in the body. The various functions of vitamin-A compounds—which include regulating growth, immunity, and the function of tumor-suppressor genes—suggest that these substances may be effective for cancer treatment. Whether natural or synthetic, vitamin-A compounds have the same chemical structure and belong to a class of substances known as *retinoids.* This substance class includes vitamin A itself (retinol and retinal), and the pharmaceuticals bexarotene (Tagretin, an approved treatment for a type of lymphoma), isotretinoin (the acne medication Accutane), and tretinoin, which is also known as all-trans retinoic acid (ATRA) or simply retinoic acid. Tretinoin is sold under brand names such as Retin-A, which is for topical use against acne, and Vesanoid, a drug specifically used for treating leukemia. Vitamin A is also related to a group of plant pigments known as *carotenoids*—10 percent of these compounds can be converted into vitamin A. Some,

including beta-carotene and lycopene (see page 121), also poss
anti-cancer properties, which is why eating foods (mostly fruits and
vegetables) that contain carotenoids is considered beneficial for cancer prevention.

When consumed in excess, vitamin A can become toxic and cause
nausea, headache, fatigue, loss of appetite, dizziness, dry skin, and
even liver damage. And although there have been many population-
based studies on vitamin A, there is still no firm evidence of its preventative or therapeutic effectiveness for cancer when used by itself.
It is best to supplement with vitamin A only when a blood test indicates a deficiency. Supplementation should always be carried out
under the supervision of a qualified healthcare professional.

VITAMIN C*

Also known as *ascorbic acid*, vitamin C is a water-soluble vitamin
obtained from food sources. It is essential for good health, functioning as an antioxidant as well as a co-factor in multiple enzyme reac-
tions needed for proper cell maintenance. In animals, vitamin C helps
heal wounds and prevents capillaries from bleeding. Vitamin-C deficiency, often caused by inadequate consumption of fresh plant foods,
can lead to a disease called *scurvy.*

Since its discovery by Hungarian scientist Albert Szent-Györgyi
in 1932, vitamin C has probably been the most intensely investigated
vitamin. Its study won Szent-Györgyi the Nobel Prize and captured
the attention of Linus Pauling, another Nobel Laureate, in his later
years. The use of vitamin C as a cancer treatment actually originates
in Pauling's hypothesis that patients treated with megadoses of vitamin C may survive longer than expected.[71] Today, there are more
than 3,000 citations for the topic "vitamin C and cancer" in the US
National Library of Medicine database.

Despite numerous studies, the usefulness and appropriate dosage
of vitamin C remain disputed. Most research has not found an obvious link between cancer prevention and vitamin C. A recent large,
randomized, double-blind, and placebo-controlled trial involving
more than 14,000 men found that vitamin C did not significantly pro-

al, lung, and prostate cancer.[72] (The dosage used
) milligrams per day taken for an average of eight
ary to Pauling's 1976 hypothesis, randomized and
:d studies by the Mayo Clinic did not find that sur-
for terminal cancer patients receiving high doses (10
grams per ᵆ of vitamin C.[73] Similarly, a review of thirty-eight studies—which looked at the effectiveness of vitamin C as both a cancer
preventative and treatment—found scant evidence that vitamin C
improves cancer survival.[74]

A study by the US National Institutes of Health in 2005, however,
had more encouraging results, which renewed interest in vitamin C
as a potential cancer treatment. The study suggested that a much
higher concentration of vitamin C in the blood—administered intra-
venously rather than orally—could have anti-cancer effects.[75] Another phase I study indicated that injecting vitamin C in doses of 1.5
grams per kilogram of body weight three times per week could have
therapeutic benefits.[76] Phase II clinical trials evaluating the effectiveness of intravenous vitamin C as a cancer treatment are currently
underway. Moreover, there is preliminary clinical evidence that, in
some cases, vitamin C may work synergistically with other anti-
cancer agents.[77]

There are some common intestinal side effects of vitamin C, especially when taken in megadoses. However, such side effects are mild
and self-limited. In general, the potential risks that are associated
with vitamin C use are not well-substantiated. For example, although
it has been widely claimed that the vitamin increases the risk of kidney stones, this link has not been confirmed by scientists. Researchers
at Sloan-Kettering have also speculated that vitamin C may promote
cancer, but this effect has not been reported in humans. In addition,
there has been concern that because it is an antioxidant, vitamin C
may reduce the effectiveness of radiation and certain chemotherapies—treatments that kill cancer cells by means of oxidative damage.
This issue is an ongoing source of controversy between the conventional and alternative medicine communities. As such, cancer
patients receiving chemotherapy or radiation treatment should be
prudent and avoid taking vitamin C supplements, especially since
there is no proven need for them.

Currently, there is not enough evidence to support the use of vitamin C as a cancer preventative or treatment at any dose. Vitamins A, D, E, and K are all better established scientifically for this purpose. Still, vitamin C may be useful when used in combination with other agents such as vitamin K (see page 134), but this decision is one best made by an experienced healthcare professional.

VITAMIN D3

The term "vitamin D" refers to several different forms of this fat-soluble vitamin, one of which is vitamin D_3. Vitamin D_3 is produced in the skin when it is exposed to the sun, and its bioactive form, *calcitriol*, is eventually activated in the liver, kidneys, and immune cells. As calcitriol, vitamin D_3 regulates calcium and bone metabolism, reduces inflammation, and affects many genes that control cell growth, which is why it's important for cancer prevention and treatment. Furthermore, many cancers contain vitamin D receptors. A number of lab experiments have demonstrated that calcitriol can inhibit the proliferation of a wide variety of cancer cells.

In 2006, Dr. Cedric F. Garland's group at the University of California conducted a review of sixty-three studies on vitamin D and cancer risk, finding that the majority had demonstrated the protective effects of vitamin D_3.[78] Garland's group suggested that an additional 1,000 international units (IU) of vitamin D_3 per day may reduce the risk of colon cancer by 50 percent.[79] There have been comparable findings reported for breast, ovarian, pancreatic, renal, and prostate cancer.[80]

One of the most robust epidemiologic studies on vitamin D_3 and cancer was conducted by Dr. Edward Giovannucci and others at the Harvard School of Public Health. Using a large group of healthy test subjects, the study found that increasing levels of 25 (OH)-cholecalciferol (a form of vitamin D_3) in the blood were associated with reduced risk of acute leukemia, as well as head and neck, esophageal, and pancreatic cancers, by more than 50 percent.[81]

In addition to cancer prevention, vitamin D_3 may also have potential as an actual cancer treatment, especially when used adjunctively with other cancer therapies. Pre-clinical testing in both animals and the laboratory has found that vitamin D_3 can work synergistically with a wide range of cancer treatments, including chemotherapy, radiation, histone deacetylase inhibitors, retinoids, tyrosine kinase inhibitors, and nonstereoidal anti-inflammatory drugs (NSAIDs).[82] Combining vitamin D_3 with other anti-cancer agents may hold promise for treating the disease, and synthetic vitamin D analogs are currently undergoing trials. However, based on a handful of phase II trials, the effectiveness of vitamin D_3 as a single-agent cancer treatment is so far disappointing. So, while there is relatively strong and consistent evidence for vitamin D_3 as a cancer preventative, its use as a cancer treatment needs to be further studied.

The recommended dosage of vitamin D_3 as a cancer preventative is in the vicinity of 2,000 to 4,000 international units (IU) per day. The exact amount should be determined with a blood test to measure the level of vitamin D3 present in the individual's body. In general, no toxicity is expected with doses below 10,000 IU or a vitamin D_3 blood level less than 150 nanograms per milliliter (ng/mL). The use of this vitamin, which must be taken with food, should be monitored by a qualified healthcare professional.

VITAMIN E

See Tocotrienols.

VITAMIN K

K ("Koagulation") vitamins are probably the most underappreciated of all the vitamin groups. They are needed mainly for blood clotting, but are also involved in bone and tissue metabolism. Vitamin K was discovered by the Danish scientist Henrik Dam, who observed blood clotting problems and abnormal bleeding in chickens fed a diet deficient in the vitamin. The fat-soluble vitamins K_1 and K_2 are found mainly in green leafy vegetables, vegetable oils, and some cereals, but are also naturally produced in the intestine. Vitamins K_3, K_4, and

K_5 are synthetic versions of the vitamin that are used in dietary supplements. However, vitamin K deficiency is unusual, so supplementation is rarely necessary for nutritional purposes.

Since the 1950s, vitamin K has been tested in test-tube and animal studies, which found that the substance can inhibit various cancers and enhance certain chemotherapy drugs. Yet, the clinical potential of vitamin K as an anti-cancer agent was recognized only recently in 2004, when a Japanese scientist discovered that women given vitamin K_2 to protect their bones cut their risk of liver cancer by 90 percent.[83] Since then, many of the studies on vitamin K and cancer have been done in Japan and have focused specifically on liver cancer. One trial showed a 30-percent drop in liver cancer recurrence when patients took vitamin K_2 supplements for three years.[84]

Although treating cancer with vitamin K alone does not always seem to prolong survival, combining the vitamin with other agents, especially vitamin C, is a promising strategy.[85] A recent trial showed that the drug Apatone, a combination of vitamins K_3 and C, slowed the progression of advanced prostate cancer. Fourteen out of the fifteen patients in the trial were still alive more than a year later and had not experienced any side effects that could be attributed to the treatment.[86] Another trial combining K_2 with an angiotensin-converting enzyme considerably reduced liver cancer recurrence.[87]

Most studies used oral dosages of vitamin K_2 and K_3 of up to 45 milligrams per day. Vitamin K_2 has not been known to cause toxicity, but side effects are possible when taking K_3, since it is synthetic. Because vitamin K may negatively interact with blood thinners such as warfarin (Coumadin), patients taking such medications should avoid use of the vitamin. Patients should take vitamin K only after consulting a qualified healthcare professional who will oversee its use.

Conclusion

Beginning my career at Memorial Sloan-Kettering Cancer Center as a junior staff member in the summer of 1987, I was at once naïve and overwhelmed—there was much to learn and little time between patient care and study. It was obvious that cancer was difficult to understand, more difficult to treat, and most difficult to cure. But at the same time, it was not easy to take a step back and reflect upon what we, as doctors, were actually doing to our patients, what cancer treatment could accomplish, and in what direction it should head. We were drilled to follow protocols, leaving little room for flexible and tailored treatment. Moreover, in many cases, we went along with the recommendations of a committee of experts or clinical practice guidelines. Like soldiers under fire, it was extremely difficult to comprehend the big picture of the war we were fighting.

So it was only very gradually that I began to question why conventional medicine's approach to cancer so often failed our patients, despite the advances being made. Time and time again over the past two decades, I have thought about how so many conventional cancer treatments are not only toxic to patients, but also ineffective. I have wondered where and why these treatments were falling short. Was it simply a lack of research and development of new drugs? Was it the slow clinical trials and bureaucratic approval process, or the high cost of cancer treatments and inadequate funding? Were doctors simply too complacent with existing treatments and established therapy protocols, and patients too stunned by their diagnosis to question their doctor's advice? Or was conventional medicine's overall approach to cancer misguided? Quite simply, was there another way?

Today, everyone continues to hope for a major breakthrough in cancer treatment, waiting for a "magic bullet" to finally win the war on cancer. But as I state early on in this book, wars are won not only with guns and firepower, but also with effective strategizing. While billions of dollars have been spent on the development of "weapons," the effort to develop a better strategy has received minimal attention. At the same time, alternative treatments—dietary supplements, diets, and mind/body approaches, for example—have been largely ignored and mistrusted due to a lack of clinical evidence, which seems to overlook one of the fundamental principles of medicine: "Do no harm." This same principle is implicit in the concept of combining various nontoxic therapies, which is part of my cultural background; Chinese medicine has taken this approach for thousands of years, and it should be seriously considered. What has not been widely considered, however, is the possibility that we already have enough "firepower." One simply has to look at the vast amount of conventional and safe alternative treatments already at our disposal. What we need is a smarter way to use the weapons we have *now*, both conventional and alternative, to fight cancer more effectively.

The idea of using a cocktail strategy to treat cancer did not come to me in a single Eureka moment, but rather occurred to me gradually. When a young breast cancer patient came to me and said, "I want to do everything I can to beat this," I realized that "doing everything" was the obvious and right thing to do. The natural answer to this patient's need was cocktail therapy—combining every possible treatment that could fight the disease effectively while minimizing harmful side effects.

Although it may not be obvious, the trend in medical research today is towards a cocktailed, multi-component, and multi-target approach, as more and more clinical trials are using combinations of agents rather than single-agent treatments. Study after study has found added benefits by combining treatment modalities and individual drugs, and drugs with non-drugs. Modern fields of science, such as network and systems biology, have created tools that will enable the discovery of more anti-cancer drug combinations.[1] Researchers are now also focused on developing new methods to assess potential synergies among cancer treatment combinations.[2] In addition, there is a separate trend towards personalized cancer therapy based on individual genetic profiling, which also sheds a hopeful light on the future of tailored anti-cancer cocktails. All of this shows how cancer treatment, as well as science in general, is gradually evolving. Little by little, we are moving beyond the search for a magic bullet.

With this said, it is important to point out the serious barriers to implementing cocktail therapy. Cancer treatment is strongly influenced—and limited—by the regulatory environment of the medical establishment, pharmaceutical companies, and health insurance providers. There is also an underlying conservatism that tends to dominate medical philosophy. Change in attitude never comes easy, and medicine is no exception. On the other hand, when something works, it is difficult to argue against it. And I am hopeful that research will continue to demonstrate the usefulness of combination treatments for cancer. Ultimately, this book is a preliminary blueprint for a different approach to cancer—an approach that I am certain will, in time, be proven by science.

I hope that this book will begin a much broader discussion of cocktail therapy among professionals and patients alike. Still, I believe that it will and must be the patients—not just physicians, researchers, the pharmaceutical industry, or the government—who will drive this discussion forward. Informed patients have much more power than they are led to believe. I hope that *Beyond the Magic Bullet* encourages patients to ask the right questions and expand their options as they continue their fight against cancer. Most of all, I hope that it helps them to overcome their disease.

In all fairness to the reader, this book could not accommodate all the discussions related to this subject. I therefore refer those who are interested in learning or contributing more to add your insights and share your opinions at the following website: www.cancercocktail.info.

Appendices

Glossary

adjunctive therapy. Another treatment used together with the primary treatment. Also called adjunct therapy, its purpose is to assist the primary treatment.

adjuvant therapy. Additional cancer treatment given after the primary treatment in order to reduce the risk of cancer recurrence. Adjuvant therapy may include chemotherapy, radiation therapy, hormone therapy, targeted therapy, and immunotherapy.

alternative medicine. Practices used instead of standard treatments that are, in general, not recognized by the medical community as standard or conventional medical approaches. Examples of alternative medicine include dietary supplements, megadose vitamins, herbal preparations, special teas, acupuncture, massage therapy, magnet therapy, spiritual healing, and meditation.

anaplasia. A term used to describe cancer cells that divide rapidly, and have little or no resemblance to normal cells.

angiogenesis. Blood vessel formation. Tumor angiogenesis refers to the growth of new blood vessels that tumors need to grow.

anti-angiogenic therapy. A type of targeted therapy that prevents the development of new blood vessels in order to block the growth of tumors.

apoptosis. A type of cell death in which a series of molecular steps in a cell leads to its death. This is the body's normal way of getting rid of unneeded or abnormal cells. The process of apoptosis may be blocked in cancer cells. Also called programmed cell death.

apoptotic therapy. A type of therapy that targets specific genes and cellular pathways involved in the process of apoptosis in order to induce the death of cancer cells.

autophagy. A normal process in which a cell destroys proteins and other substances in its cytoplasm (the fluid inside the cell membrane but outside the nucleus), which may lead to cell death. Autophagy may prevent normal cells from developing into cancer cells, but it may also protect cancer cells by destroying anti-cancer drugs or substances taken up by them.

brachytherapy. A type of radiation therapy in which radioactive material is sealed in needles, seeds, wires, or catheters, and placed directly into or near a tumor. Also called implant radiation therapy, internal radiation therapy, and radiation brachytherapy.

cauterization. The process by which tissue is destroyed using a hot or cold instrument, an electrical current, or a chemical that burns or dissolves the tissue. This ancient method may still be used to kill certain types of small tumors.

cell differentiation. The process by which young, immature (unspecialized) cells take on individual characteristics and reach their mature (specialized) form and function.

chemotherapy. Treatment with drugs that kill cancer cells. Combination chemotherapy involves the use of more than one anti-cancer drug.

clinical trial. A type of research study that tests how well new medical approaches work in people. These studies test new methods of screening, prevention, diagnosis, or treatment of a disease. Also called clinical study.

cryosurgery. Also called cryoablation and cryosurgical ablation, this is a minimally invasive cryotherapy that destroys abnormal cells by freezing the tissue with liquid nitrogen, carbon dioxide, or argon gas.

cryotherapy. Term used to describe any therapy that uses cold temperature to treat cancer.

curative surgery. Removal of an entire tumor with the intent of curing the cancer.

cyclin-dependent kinases (CDKs). A group of proteins instrumental in regulating cell growth. An imbalance of these proteins is associated with most cancers, making CDKs a potential target for cancer treatment.

cytokines. A chemical messenger produced by cells of the immune system. Some cytokines can boost the immune response, while others can suppress it. Cytokines can also be made in the laboratory by recombinant DNA technology and used in the treatment of cancer, among other diseases.

cytotoxicity. Causing cell death.

debulking surgery. Surgical removal of as much of a tumor as possible. Debulking may increase the chance that chemotherapy or radiation therapy will kill all the tumor cells. Also called tumor debulking, this procedure may also be done to relieve symptoms or extend the survival time of the patient.

diagnostic surgery. Removal of cancerous tissue in order to analyze it and determine the type, as well as the stage, of the cancer. Also called staging surgery.

drug interaction. A change in the way a drug acts in the body when taken with certain other drugs, herbs, or foods, or when taken with certain medical conditions. Drug interactions may cause a drug to become more or less effective, or produce unexpected effects in the body.

dysplasia. A condition in which cells look abnormal under a microscope but are not cancerous.

epigenetic therapy. Refers to a new type of therapy aimed at affecting gene expression (i.e., the turning "on" and "off" of genes) in order to inhibit the growth of cancer or affect the course of the disease.

hormone therapy. Treatment that adds, blocks, or removes hormones. To slow or stop the growth of certain cancers (such as prostate and breast cancer), synthetic hormones or other drugs may be given to block the body's production of natural hormones. Sometimes surgery is needed to remove the gland that makes a certain hormone. This therapy is also referred to as endocrine therapy, hormonal therapy, and hormone treatment.

hyperplasia. An abnormal increase in the number of normal cells in an organ or tissue.

hyperthermia therapy. A type of treatment in which body tissue is exposed to high temperatures in order to damage and kill cancer cells, or to make cancer cells more sensitive to the effects of radiation and certain anti-cancer drugs.

immunotherapy. Treatment that enhances or restores the ability of the immune system to fight cancer, infections, and other diseases. It is also used to lessen certain side effects that may be caused by some cancer treatments. Agents used in immunotherapy include monoclonal antibodies, growth factors, and vaccines. These agents may also have a direct anti-tumor effect. Also called biological response modifier therapy, biological therapy, biotherapy, and BRM therapy.

intensity-modulated radiation therapy (IMRT). A type of conformal radiation therapy that uses computer-generated images to outline a tumor's shape and size. By changing the intensity of radiation during treatment, the damage to surrounding healthy tissue is reduced.

interferon. A biological response modifier, which is a substance that can improve the body's natural response to infections and other diseases. Interferons disrupt the division of cancer cells and can slow tumor growth. There are several types of interferons, including interferon-alpha, -beta, and -gamma, that are normally produced by the body. Interferons are also made in the laboratory to treat cancer and other diseases.

laparoscopic surgery. Surgery done with the aid of a laparoscope, which is a thin, tube-like instrument with a light and a lens for viewing. It may also have a tool designed to remove tissue to be checked under a microscope for signs of disease. Also called laparoscopic-assisted resection.

laser surgery. A surgical procedure that uses the cutting power of a laser beam to make bloodless cuts in tissue or remove a surface lesion such as a tumor.

male hormone (androgen) ablation. Treatment that suppresses or blocks the production or action of male hormones. This may involve the removal of the testicles, or taking female sex hormones or drugs called antiandrogens. Also called androgen deprivation and androgen suppression.

microscopically controlled surgery. A technique for removing certain cancerous tumors based on careful and precise microscopic control of the surgical margins, or the border of tissue surrounding the tumor. Originally conceived and implemented by Frederic Mohs, this procedure is also called Mohs surgery and chemosurgery.

microsphere therapy. This type of treatment involves the injection of microspheres—tiny, hollow, round particles made from materials such as glass, ceramic, or plastic—into blood vessels that feed a tumor to cut off its blood supply. Microspheres can also be filled with a substance (for example, radiation) that may help kill more cancer cells. Specialized types of this therapy include SIR-Sphere and TheraSphere.

molecular pathway. A series of actions among molecules in a cell that leads to a certain end point or cell function.

monotherapy. A term used to describe a type of therapy, usually a drug, used by itself. Monotherapy is generally the approach taken when a single medication or other treatment is sufficient to treat or cure a particular condition.

multidimensional conformal radiotherapy. A specialized radiation treatment in which radiologic imaging and computer technology is used to match the beams of radiation to the size and shape of the tumor. A similar technique is known as three-dimensional conformal radiation therapy (3DCRT).

multidrug resistance (MDR). Adaptation of tumor cells to anti-cancer drugs in ways that make the drugs less effective.

off-label. A legal term describing the use of a pharmaceutical drug to treat a condition other than that for which the drug is approved by the US Food and Drug Administration and similar health authorities.

oncolytic virus therapy. A type of targeted therapy using a special type of virus that infects and breaks down cancer cells, but not normal cells. This therapy may make it easier to kill tumor cells with chemotherapy and radiation therapy. It is also referred to as oncolytic virotherapy, viral therapy, and virotherapy.

palliative surgery. An operation intended to alleviate and control the symptoms of cancer, such as pain, rather than treat the disease itself.

P-glycoprotein (P-gp). A protein that pumps substances out of cells. Cancer cells that have too much P-glycoprotein may be able to push out anti-cancer drugs directed at them, thereby rendering the drugs ineffective.

photodynamic therapy. Treatment with drugs that become active when exposed to light. These activated drugs may kill cancer cells.

preventive surgery. Surgery performed to reduce the likelihood of cancer development by removing the organ at risk, such as the breasts or ovaries.

proton beam radiation therapy. A type of radiation therapy that uses streams of protons that are emitted from a special machine. This type of radiation kills tumor cells but does not damage nearby tissues. It is used to treat cancers in the head and neck, and in organs such as the brain, eye, lung, spine, and prostate. Proton beam radiation is different from x-ray radiation.

proto-oncogene. A gene involved in normal cell growth. Mutations in a proto-oncogene may cause it to become an oncogene, which can cause the growth of cancer cells.

radiation therapy (radiation). The use of high-energy radiation from x-rays, gamma rays, neutrons, protons, and other sources to kill cancer cells and shrink tumors. Radiation may come from a machine outside the body (external-beam radiation therapy), or it may come from radioactive material placed in the body near cancer cells (internal radiation therapy). Systemic radiation therapy uses a radioactive substance, such as a radiolabeled monoclonal antibody, that travels in the blood to tissues throughout the body. Also called radiotherapy.

radiofrequency ablation (RFA). A procedure that uses radio waves to heat and destroy abnormal cells. This technique, which can be effective even for cancers deep within an organ, is being used increasingly for liver tumors, and may be applied to lung and bone cancers as well.

radioimmunotherapy. A type of systemic radiation therapy in which a radioactive substance is linked to an antibody that locates and kills tumor cells when injected into the body.

reductionism. An approach to understanding complex ideas or entities by reducing them to their simpler individual components. This philosophy is based on the principle that all things are the sum of their parts.

robotic surgery. Surgical procedure performed with the aid of a robotic system controlled by a computer.

signal transduction inhibitor. A substance that blocks signals passed from one molecule to another inside a cell. Blocking these signals can affect many functions of the cell, including cell division and cell death, and may kill cancer cells. Certain signal transduction inhibitors are being studied in the treatment of cancer.

sonodynamic therapy. An experimental treatment that uses ultrasound to boost the cytotoxic effects of special drugs known as sonosensitizers.

stereotactic radiosurgery. A type of external radiation therapy that uses special equipment to position the patient and precisely administer a single large dose of radiation to a tumor. It is used to treat brain tumors and other brain disorders that cannot be treated by regular surgery. It is also being studied in the treatment of other types of cancer. Also called radiation surgery and stereotaxic radiosurgery, specific types of this procedure include CyberKnife and Gamma Knife.

synergy. In medicine, a term used to describe the interaction of two or more drugs when their combined effect is greater than the sum of the effects observed when each drug is given alone.

systemic radiation therapy. A type of radiation therapy in which a radioactive substance, such as radioactive iodine or a radioactively labeled monoclonal antibody, is swallowed or injected into the body and travels through the blood, locating and killing tumor cells.

targeted therapy. A type of treatment that uses drugs or other substances, such as monoclonal antibodies, to identify and attack specific cancer cells. Targeted therapy may have fewer side effects than other types of cancer treatments.

Traditional Chinese Medicine (TCM). A medical system that has been used for thousands of years to prevent, diagnose, and treat disease. It is based in part on the belief that qi (the body's vital energy) flows along meridians (channels) throughout the body and keeps a person's spiritual, emotional, mental, and physical health in balance. Traditional Chinese Medicine aims to restore the body's balance and harmony between the natural opposing forces of yin and yang, which can block qi and cause disease. TCM includes acupuncture, diet, herbal therapy, meditation, physical exercise, and massage.

transarterial chemoembolization (TACE). A two-step therapy used in the treatment of liver cancer. Chemotherapy drugs are directly administered to the tumor via the artery that supplies blood to the liver, effectively targeting the cancer while avoiding side effects associated with whole-body chemotherapy. Following this treatment, the blood supply to the tumor is embolized, or cut off.

tumor suppressor gene. A type of gene that makes a protein called a tumor suppressor protein that helps control cell growth. Mutations in these genes may lead to cancer. Also called anti-oncogene.

tumor surveillance theory. A theory conceived by Dr. Thomas Lewis and Dr. McFarlane Burnet in the 1950s, it proposes that the human immune system has specialized white blood cells that locate and destroy cancer cells. This theory sparked interest in the relationship between cancer and the immune system, and ultimately led to the development of immunotherapy.

References

Introduction

1. Ho, D. "Discovering the HIV/AIDS Drug 'Cocktail' in an Equation." Transcript. May 2, 2010. http://bigthink.com/ideas/19910.

2. Williams, B. *Surviving Terminal Cancer: Clinical Trials, Drug Cocktails, and Other Treatments Your Oncologist Won't Tell You About.* Minneapolis, MN: Fairview Press, 2002.

PART 1: THE BIOLOGY AND TREATMENT OF CANCER

Chapter 1

1. Abbott, RG, et al. "Simulating the hallmarks of cancer." *Artificial Life* 2006; 12(4):613–634.

2. Grizzi, F, Chiriva-Internati, M. "Cancer: Looking for simplicity and finding complexity." *Cancer Cell Int.* 2006;6:4.

3. National Cancer Institute. "Integrative cancer biology program: Tackling cancer's complexity." *NCI Cancer Bulletin* 2005; 1(8):5.

4. Weinberg, RA. *One Renegade Cell.* New York: Basic Books, 1998.

5. Fox, M. "Study details complexity of cancer—sheds light on difficulty of cure." *Reuters.* September 5, 2008.

Chapter 2

1. Coley, WB. "The treatment of malignant tumors by repeated inoculations of erysipelas. With a report of ten original cases." 1893. *Clin Orthop* 1991; 262:3–11.

2. Weiner, LM. "Immunotherapy for cancer—the endgame begins." *NEJM* 2008; 358:2664–2665.

3. Folkman, J. "Successful treatment of an angiogenic disease." *NEJM* 1989; 320(18):1211–1212.

4. Santos, FP, et al. "Decitabine in the treatment of myelodysplastic syndromes." *Expert Rev Anticancer Ther.* 2010 10(1):9–22.

Chapter 3

1. Scheid, V, et al. *Chinese Herbal Medicine: Formulas & Strategies.* Seattle, WA: Eastland Press, 2009.

2. Sugland, B, et al. "Impact of zidovudine and other factors on the natural history of AIDS." *Int Conf AIDS* 1990, June 20–23; 6:435. Abstract no. 3132.

Chapter 4

1. Keith, CT, et al. "Mutlicomponent therapeutics for networked systems." *Nat Rev Drug Discov* 2005; 4:71–78.

2. Shewach, DS, et al. "Antimetabolite radiosensitizers." *J Clin Oncol* 2007; 25(26):4043–4050.

3. Burke, PA, DeNardo, SJ. "Antiangiogenic agents and their promising potential in combined therapy." *Oncol Hematol* 2001; 39(1–2):155–171

4. Baxevanis, CN, et al. "Combinatorial treatments including vaccines, chemotherapy, and monoclonal antibodies for cancer therapy." *Cancer Immunol Immunother* 2009; 58(3):317–324.

5. Gough, MJ, Crittenden, MR. "Combination approaches to immunotherapy: the radiotherapy example." *Immunotherapy* 2009; 1(6):1025–1037.

6. Kamrava, M, et al. "Combining radiation, immunotherapy, and antiangiogenesis agent in the management of cancer." *Mol Biosyst* 2009; 5(11): 1262–1270.

7. De Schutter, H, Nuyts, S. "Radiosensitizing potential of epigenetic cancer drugs." *Anticancer Agents Med Chem* 2009; 9(1):99–108.

8. O'Reagan, B, Hirshberg, C. *Spontaneous Remissions — An Annotated Bibliography.* Petaluma, CA: Inst. Of Noetic Sciences, 1993.

9. Nobili, S, et al. "Pharmacological strategies for overcoming multidrug resistance." *Curr Drug Targets* 2006; 7(7):861–879.

10. Bansal T, et al. Emerging significance of flavonoids as P-glycoprotein inhibitors in cancer. *J Pharm Pharm Sci* 2009;12(1): 46–78.

11. Wong, CM, et al. "Clinically significant drug-drug interactions between oral anticancer agents: profiling and comparison of two drug compendia." *Ann Pharmacother* 2008; 42(12):1737–1748.

12. Beer, TM, Myrthue, A. "Calcitriol in cancer treatment: from the lab to the clinic." *Mol Cancer Ther* 2004; 3(3):373–381.

13. Verrax, J, Calderon, PB. The controversial place of vitamin C in cancer treatment. *Biochem Pharmacol* 2008; 76(12): 1644-52, 2008.

14. Block K, et al. Impact of antioxidant supplementation on chemotherapeutic efficacy: a systematic review of the evidence from randomized controlled trials. *Cancer Treat Rev* 2007; 33(5):407–18. 2007.

15. DiMasi, JA, et al. "The price of innovation: new estimates of drug development costs." *J Health Econ* 2003; 22:151–185.

16. Freireich, EJ, et al. "Quadruple combination therapy (VAMP) for acute lymphocytic leukemia of childhood." *Pro Am Assoc Cancer Res* 1964; 5:20.

17. Winter, MC, Hancock, BW. "Ten years of rituximab in NHL." *Expert Opin Drug Saf* 2009; 8(2):223–235.

Chapter 5

1. Shewach, DS, Lawrence, TS. "Antimetabolite radiosensitizers." *J Clin Oncol* 2007; 25(26):4043–4050.

2. Burke, PA, DeNardo, SJ. "Antiangiogenic agents and their promising potential in combined therapy." *Oncol Hematol* 2001; 39(1–2):155–171.

3. Baxevanis, CN, Perez, SA, Papamichail, M. "Combinatorial treatments including vaccines, chemotherapy and monoclonal antibodies for cancer therapy." *Cancer Immunol Immonther* 2009; 58(3):317–324.

4. Gough, MJ, Crittenden, MR. "Combination approaches to immunotherapy: the radiotherapy example." *Immunotherapy* 2009; 1(6):1025–1037.

5. Kamrava, M, et al. "Combining radiation, immunotherapy, and antiangiogenesis agents in the management of cancer" *Mol Biosyst* 2009; 5(11):1262–1270.

6. De Schutter, H, Nuyts, S. "Radiosensitizing potential of epigenetic anticancer drugs." *Anticancer Agents Med Chem* 2009; 9(1):99–108.

7. Richardson, PG, et al. "Lenalidomide, bortezomib, and dexamethasone combination therapy in patients with newly diagnosed multiple myeloma." *Blood* 2010; 116(5):679–686.

8. Dana-Farber/ Harvard Cancer Center. "Bench to bedside translational science doubling myeloma survival." http://www.dfhcc.harvard.edu/news/ announcements/article/3062/185/.

9. Interactive European Network for Industrial Crops and their Applications 2000–2005. "Summary Report for the European Union." http://www.ienica.net/reports/ienicafinalsummaryreport2000-2005.pdf.

10. Campbell, TC, Campbell, TM. *The China Study: The Most Comprehensive Study of Nutrition Ever Conducted and the Startling Implications for Diet, Weight Loss, and Long-term Health.* Dallas, TX: BenBella Books, 2006.

11. Doll, R, Peto, R. "The causes of cancer: Quantitative estimates of avoidable risks of cancer in the United States today." *J Natl Cancer Ins* 1981; 66:1191–1308.

12. Moreschi, C. "Beziehungen zwischen ernahrung und tumorwachstum." *Z. fur Immunitatsforsch* 1909; 2:651–675.

13. McCay, CM, Crowell, MF. "Prolonging the Life Span." *The Scientific Monthly* 1934; 39(5):405–414.

14. Hursting, SD, et al. "Calories and carcinogenesis: lessons learned from 30 years of calorie restriction research." *Carcinogenesis* 2010; 31(1):83–89.

15. Cleman, RJ, et al. "Caloric restriction delays disease onset and mortality in rhesus monkeys." *Science* 2009; 325(5937):201–204.

16. Kushi, M. "A cancer approach from dietetics according to the principles of macrobiotics." *Farm Tijdschr Belg* 1979; 56:353–358.

17. Carter, JP, et al. "Hypothesis: dietary management may improve survival from nutritionally linked cancers based on analysis of representative cases." *J Am Coll Nutr* 1993; 12:209–226.

18. Kelly, WD, Rohe, F. *Cancer: Curing the Incurable Without Surgery, Chemotherapy, or Radiation* Bonita, CA: New Century Promotions, 2000.

19. Frankl, V. *Man's Search for Meaning.* Boston: Beacon Press, 1959; Reprint, 2006.

20. LeShan, L. *Cancer As a Turning Point: A Handbook for People with Cancer, Their Families, and Health Professionals.* New York: Plume, 1994.

21. Godbout, JP, and Glaser, R. "Stress-induced immune dysregulation: implications for wound healing, infectious disease, and cancer." *J Neuroimmune Pharmacol* 2006; 1(4):421–427.

22. Anderson, BL, et al. "Biobehavioral, immune, and health benefits following recurrence for psychological intervention participants." *Clin Cancer Res* 2010; 16(12):3270–3278.

Chapter 6

1. Bendapudi, NM, et al. "Patients perspectives on ideal physician behaviors." *Mayo Clinic Proc* 2006; 81(3):338–344.

2. Allison, M. "Trouble at the office." *Nat Biotechnol* 2008; 26(9):967–969.

3. Kolata, G, Pollack, A. "The Evidence Gap—Costly Cancer Drug Offers Hope, but Also a Dilemma." *The New York Times.* Jul 6, 2008.

4. Editorial. "When a Drug Fails." *The New York Times.* Jul 25, 2010.

5. Markel, H. "Supply-Side Oncology." *The New York Times.* Feb 4, 2001.

6. Kowal, CD, Bertino, JR. "Possible benefits of hyperthermia to chemotherapy." *Cancer Res* 1979; 39(6 Pt 2):2285–2289.

7. Loverock, P, ter Haar, T. "Synergism between hyperthermia, ultrasound, and gamma irradiation." *Ultrasound Med Biol* 1991; 17)6):607–612.

8. Patel, BB, Majumdar, AP. "Synergistic role of curcumin with current therapeutics in colorectal cancer: minireview." *Nutr Cancer* 2009; 61(6):842–846.

9. Zhang, X, et al. "Synergistic inhibition of head and neck tumor growth by green tea (-)-epigallocatechin-3-gallate and EGFR tyrosine kinase inhibitor." *Int J Cancer* 2008; 123(5):1005–1014.

10. Casado-Zapico, S, et al. "Synergistic antitumor effect of melatonin with several chemotherapeutic drugs on human Ewing sarcoma cancer cells: potentiation of the extrinsic apoptotic pathway." *J Pineal Res* 2010; 48(1):72–80.

11. Kenny, FS, et al. "Effect of dietary GLA + / -tamoxifen on the growth, ER expression, and fatty acid profile of ER positive human breast cancer xenografts." *Int J Cancer* 2001; 92(3):342–347.

12. Zee-Cheng, RK. "Shi-quan-da-bu-tang (ten significant tonic decoction), SQT. A potent Chinese biological response modifier in cancer immunotherapy, potentiation and detoxification of anticancer drugs." *Methods Find Exp Clin Pharmacol* 1992; 14(9):725–736.

13. Chung, VQ, et al. "Interactions of a herbal combination that inhibits growth of prostate cancer cells." *Cancer Chemother Pharmacol* 2004; 53(5):384–390.

14. Calderon, PB, et al. "Potential therapeutic application of the association of vitamins C and K_3 in cancer treatment." *Curr Med Chem* 2002; 9(24):2271–2285.

15. Wiginton, DP, et al. "Combination study of 1,24(S)-dihydroxyvitamin D2 and chemotherapeutic agents on human breast and prostate cancer cell lines." *Anticancer Res* 2004; 24(5A):2905–2912.

16. Koren, R, et al. "Synergistic anticancer activity of 1,25-dihydroxyvitamin D(3) and immune cytokines: the involvement of reactive oxygen species." *J Steroid Biochem Mol Biol* 2000; 73(3–4):105–112.

17. Hilakivi-Clarke, L, et al. "Is soy consumption good or bad for the breast?" *J Nutr* Oct 27, 2010.

18. Iarussi, D, et al. "Protective effect of coenzyme Q_{10} on anthracyclines cardiotoxicity: control study in children with acute lymphoblastic leukemia and non-Hodgkin lymphoma." *Mol Aspects* 2004; 15 (Suppl):s207–212.

19. Lissoni, P. "Biochemotherapy with standard chemotherapies plus the pineal hormone melatonin in the treatment of advanced solid neoplasms." *Pathol Biol* (Paris) 2007; 55(3–4):201–204.

20. Tan, AD, et al. "A patient-level meta-analytic investigation of the prognostic significance of baseline quality of life (QOL) for overall survival (OS) among 3,704 patients participating in 24 North Central Cancer Treatment Group (NCCTG) and Mayo Clinic Cancer Center (MC) oncology clinical trials." *J Clin Oncol* 2008; 26 (May 20 suppl; abstr 9515).

21. Quinten, C, et al. "Baseline quality of life as a prognostic indicator of survival: a meta-analysis of individual patient data from EORTC clinical trials." *Lancet Oncol* 2009; 10(9):865–871.

OFF-LABEL DRUGS AND DIETARY SUPPLEMENTS LISTS

Off-Label Drugs

1. Armitage, JO, Sidner, RD. "Anti-tumor effect of cimetidine." *Lancet* 1979; 1(8121):882–883.

2. Mentz, F, et al. "Theophylline, a new inducer of apoptosis in B-CLL: Role of cyclic nucleotides." *Br J Haematol* 1995; 90(4):957–959.

3. Wiernik, PH, et al. "Phase II study of theophylline in chronic lymphocytic leukemia: a study of the Eastern Cooperative Oncology Group (E4998)." *Leukemia* 2004; 18(10):1605–1610.

4. Willis, CR, et al. "A phase I / II study examining pentostatin, chlorambucil, and theophylline in patients with relapsed chronic lymphocytic leukemia and non-Hodgkin's lymphoma." *Ann Hematol* 2006; 85(5):301–307.

5. Sassa, R, et al. "Differential modulating effects of clarithromycin on the production of cytokines by a tumor." *Antimicrob Agents Chemother* 1999; 43:787–789.

6. Coleman, M, et al. "BLT-D (clarithromycin [Biaxin], low-dose thalidomide, and dexamethasone) for the treatment of myeloma and Waldenström's macroglobulinemia." *Leuk Lymphoma* 2002; 43(9):1777–1782.

7. Niesvizky, R, et al. "BiRD (Biaxin [clarithromycin] / Revlimid [lenalidomide] / dexamethasone) combination therapy results in high complete—and overall—response rates in treatment-naive symptomatic multiple myeloma." *Blood* 2008; 111(3):1101–1109.

8. Gay, F, et al. "Clarithromycin (Biaxin)-lenalidomide-low-dose dexamethasone (BiRD) versus lenalidomide-low-dose dexamethasone (Rd) for newly diagnosed myeloma." *Am J Hematol* 2010; 85(9):664–669.

9. Mikasa, K, et al. "Significant survival benefit to patients with advanced non-small cell lung cancer from treatment with clarithromycin." *Chemotherapy* 1997; 43(4):288–296.

10. Kamat, AM, et al. "Quinolone antibiotics: a potential adjunct to intravesical chemotherapy for bladder cancer." *Urology* 1999; 54(1):56–61.

11. Tagalakis, V, et al. "Use of warfarin and risk of urogenital cancer: a population-based, nested case-control study." *Lancet Oncol* 2007; 8(5):395–402.

12. Akl, EA, et al. "Oral anticoagulation may prolong survival of a subgroup of patients with cancer: a Cochrane systematic review." *J Exp Clin Cancer Res* 2007; 26(2):175–184.

13. Mousa, SA, Petersen, LJ. "Anti-cancer properties of low-molecular-weight heparin: preclinical evidence." *Thromb Haemost* 2009; 102(2):258–267.

14. Icli, F, et al. "Low molecular weight heparin (LMWH) increases the efficacy of cisplatinum plus gemcitabine combination in advanced pancreatic cancer." *J Surg Oncol* 2007; 95(6):507–512.

15. Akl, EA, et al. "Parenteral anticoagulation for prolonging survival in patients with cancer who have no other indication for coagulation." *Cochrane Database Syst Rev* 2007; 18(3):CD006652.

16. Beaney, RP, Gullan, RW, Pilkington, GJ. "Therapeutic potential of antidepressants in malignant glioma: a clinical experience with clomipramine." *J Clin Oncol* 2005; 23(16S):1535.

17. Levkovitz, Y, et al. "Differential induction of apoptosis by antidepressants in glioma and neuroblastoma cell lines: evidence for p-c-Jun, cytochrome c, and caspase-3 involvement." *J Mol Neurosci* 2005; 27(1):29–42.

18. Kebebew, E, et al. "Thyroid. Results of rosiglitazone therapy in patients with thyroglobulin-positive and radioiodine-negative advanced differentiated thyroid cancer." *Thyroid* 2009; 19(9):953–956.

19. Hau, P, et al. "Low-dose chemotherapy in combination with COX-2 inhibitors and PPAR-gamma agonists in recurrent high-grade gliomas—a phase II study." *Oncology* 2007; 73(1–2):21–25.

20. Pollack, MN. "Insulin, insulin-like growth factors, insulin resistance and neoplasia." *Am J Clin Nutri* 2007; 86(2):S820–822.

21. Libby, G, et al. "New users of metformin are at low risk of incident cancer: a cohort study among people with type 2 diabetes." *Diabetes Care* 2009; 32(9):1620–1625.

22. Jiralerspong, S, et al. "Metformin and pathologic complete responses to neoadjuvant chemotherapy in diabetic patients with breast cancer." *J Clin Oncol* 2009; 27(20):3297–3302.

23. Liebertz, C, Fox, P. "Ketoconazole as a secondary hormonal intervention in advanced prostare cancer." *Clin J Oncol Nurs* 2006; 10(3):361–366.

24. Scholz, M, et al. "Long-term outcome for men with androgen independ-

ent prostate cancer treated with ketoconazole and hydrocortisone." *J Urol* 2005; 173(6):1947–1952.

25. Flossman, E, et al. "Effect of aspirin on long-term risk of colorectal cancer: consistent evidence from randomised and observational studies." *Lancet* 2007; 369(9573):1603–1613.

26. Holmes, MD, et al. "Aspirin intake and survival after breast cancer." *J Clin Oncol* 2010; 28(9):1467–1472.

27. Chan, AT, et al. "Aspirin use and survival after diagnosis of colorectal cancer." *JAMA* 2009; 302(6):649–658.

28. Bertagnoli, MM, et al. "Celecoxib for the prevention of sporadic colorectal adenomas." *N Engl J Med* 2006; 355(9):873–884.

29. Harris, RE. "Cyclooxygenase-2 (cox-2) blockcase in the chemoprevention of cancers of the colon, breast, prostate, and lung." *Inflammopharmacology* 2009; 17(2)55–67.

30. Altorki, NK, et al. "Celecoxib, a selective cyclo-oxygenase-2 inhibitor, enhances the response to preoperative paclitaxel and carboplatin in early-stage non-small-cell-lung cancer." *Clin Oncol* 2003; 21(14):2645–2650.

31. Falandry, C, et al. "Celecoxib and exemestane versus placebo and exemestane in postmenopausal metastatic breast cancer patients: a double-blind phase III GINECO study." *Breast Cancer Res Treat* 2009; 116(3):501–508.

32. Sotelo, J, et al. "Adding chloroquine to conventional treatment for glioblastoma multiforme: a randomized, double-blind, placebo-controlled trial." *Ann Intern Med* 2006; 144(5):337–343.

33. Berger, TG, et al. "Artesunate in the treatment of metastatic uveal melanoma—first experiences." *Oncol Rep* 2005; 14(6):1599–1603.

34. Zhang, ZY, et al. "Artesunate combined with vinorelbine plus cisplaitn in treatment of advanced non-small cell lung cancer: a randomized controlled trial." [Chinese] *Zhong Xi Yi Jie He Xue Bao* 2008; 6(2):134–138.

35. The European Stroke Prevention Study (ESPS). "Principal end-points." *Lancet* 1987; 2(8572):1351–1354.

36. Rhodes, EH, et al. "Dipyridamole for treatment of melanoma." *Lancet* 1987; 2(8572):1351–1354).

37. Kohnoe, S, et al. "Treatment of advanced gastric cancer with 5-fluorouracil and cisplatin in combination with dipyridamole." *Int J Oncol* 1998; 13(6):1203–1206.

38. Todd, KE, et al. "Resection of locally advanced pancreatic cancer after downstaging with continuous-infusion-5-fluorouracil, mitomycin-C, leucovorin, and dipyridamole." *J Gastrointest Surg* 1998; 2(2):159–166.

39. Taoka, H, et al. "Adjuvant chemotherapy for unresectable locally advanced pancreatic cancer in light of its characteristics." [Japanese] *Gan To Kagaku Ryoho* 2004; 31(9):1365–1370.

40. Kuendgen, A, et al. "Results of a phase-2 study of valproic acid alone or in combination with all-trans retinoic acid in 75 patients with myelodysplastic syndrome and relapsed or refractory acute myeloid leukemia." *Ann Hematol* 2005; 84 Suppl 1:61–66.

41. Weller, M, et al. "Prolonged survival with valproic acid use in the EORTC/NCIC temozolomide trial for glioblastoma." *Neurology* 2011 August 21.

42. Bobustuc, GC, et al. "Levetiracetam enhances p53-mediated MGMT inhibition and sensitizes glioblastoma cells to temozolomide." *Neuro Oncol* 2010; 12(9): 917–927.

43. Ke, Y, et al. "Noscapine inhibits tumor growth with little toxicity to normal tissues or inhibition of immune responses." *Cancer Immunol Immunother* 2000; 49(4–5):217–225.

44. Diel, IJ, et al. "Reduction in new metastases in breast cancer with adjuvant clodronate treatment." *N Engl J Med* 1998; 339(6):357–363.

45. Powles, T, et al. "Reduction in bone relapse and improved survival with oral clodronate for adjuvant treatment of operable breast cancer." *Breast Cancer Res* 2006; 8(2):R13.

46. Chiplunkar, S, et al. "Gammadelta T cells in cancer immunotherapy: current status and future prospects." *Immunotherapy* 2009; 1(4):663–678.

47. Dieli, F, et al. "Targeting human gamma-delta T cells with zoledronate and interleukin-2 for immunotherapy of hormone-refractory prostate cancer." *Curr Opin Investig Drugs* 2008; 9(10):1089–1094.

48. Madrid, C, et al. "Bisphosphonate-related osteonecrosis of the jaws: how to manage cancer patients." *Oral Oncol* 2010; 46(6):468–470.

49. Belopomme, D, et al. "Verapamil increases the survival of patients with anthracycline-resistant metastatic breast carcinoma." *Ann Oncol* 2000; 11(11):1471–1476.

50. Naito, S, et al. "Prophylactic intravesical instillation chemotherapy against recurrence after transurethral resection of superficial bladder cancer: a randomized controlled trial of doxorubicin plus verapamil versus doxorubicin alone." *Cancer Chemother Pharmacol* 1998; 42(5):367–372.

51. Khontoghiorghes, GJ, et al. "Chelators controlling metal metabolism and toxicity pathways: applications in cancer prevention, diagnosis and treatment." *Hemoglobin* 2008; 32(1–2):217–227.

52. Kovacevic, Z, et al. "Iron chelators: development of novel compounds

with high and selective anti-tumour activity." *Curr Drug Deliv* 2010. [Epub ahead of print.]

53. Khan, G, Merajver, S. "Copper chelation in cancer therapy using tetrathiomolybdate: an evolving paradigm." *Expert Opin Investig Drugs* 2009; 18(4):541–548.

54. Berkson, BM, et al. "Revisiting the ALA/N (alpha-lipoic acid/low-dose naltrexone) protocol for people with metastatic and nonmetastatic pancreatic cancer: a report of 3 new cases." *Integr Cancer Ther* 2009; 8(4):416–422.

55. Berkson, BM. "Reversal of signs and symptoms of B-cell lymphoma in a patient using only low-dose naltrexone." *Integr Cancer Ther* 2007; 6(3):293–296.

56. Jasińska, M, et al. "Statins: a new insight into their mechanisms of action and consequent pleiotropic effects." *Pharmacol Rep* 2007; 59(5):483–499.

57. Sassano, A, Platanias, LC. "Statins in tumour suppression." *Cancer Letters* 2008; 260(1–2):11–19.

58. Poynter, JN, et al. "Statins and the risk of colorectal cancer." *New England J Med* 2005; 352:2184–2192.

59. Kocchar, R, et al. "Statins reduce breast cancer risk: A case control study in US female veterans." *J Clin Oncol* 2005; 23:7S [suppl, abstr 514].

60. Khurana, V, et al. "Statins reduce the risk of lung cancer in humans: a large case-control study of US veterans." *Chest* 2007; 131:1282–1288.

61. El-Serag, HB, et al. "Statins are associated with a reduced risk of hepatocellular carcinoma in a large cohort of patients with diabetes." *Gastroenterology* 2009; 136(5):1601–1608.

62. Murtola, TJ, et al. "Prostate cancer and PSA among statin users in the Finnish prostate cancer screening trial." *Int J Cancer* 2010 Jan 13.

63. Kawata, et al. "Effect of pravastatin on survival in patients with advanced hepatocellular carcinoma: A randomized controlled trial." *Br J Cancer* 2001; 84(7):886–891.

64. Efraim, B, et al. "Immunopotentiation and immunotherapeutic effects of thymic hormones and factors with special emphasis on thymic humoral factor THF-gamma2." *Crit Rev Immunol* 1999; 19(4):261–284.

65. Tutill, C, et al. "Thymosin alpha 1: clinical experience and future promise." *Ann NY Acad Sci* 2010; 1193:130–135.

66. Salvati, F, et al. "Combined treatment with thymosin-alpha 1 and low dose interferon-alpha after Ifosfamide in non small cell lung cancer: a phase II controlled trial." *Anticancer Res* 1996; 16(2):1001–1004.

67. Maio, M, et al. "Large randomized study of thymosin alpha 1, interferon

alpha, or both in combination with dacarbazine in patients with metastatic melanoma." *J Clin Oncol* 2010; 28(10):1780–1787.

68. Gish, RG, et al. "A randomized controlled trial of thymalfasin plus transarterial chemoembolization for unresectable hepatocellular carcinoma." *Hepatol Int* 2009 May 8.

69. Moviglia, GA, et al. "Clinical response of patients with advanced breast cancer treated with dendritic cell vaccine with and without Thymalfasin." [Abstract] *J Clin Oncology* 2005; 23:16S:2593.

Dietary Supplements

1. "Special Report: A health fad that's hard to swallow." *New Scientist*. Apr 12, 2004.

2. Cho, WC, Leung, KN. "In vitro and in vivo immunomodulating and immunorestorative effects of Astralgalus membranaceus." *J Ethnopharmacol* 2007; 113(1):132–141.

3. McCulloch, M, et al. "Astragalus-based Chinese herbs and platinum-based chemotherapy for advanced non-small-cell lung cancer: meta-analysis of randomized trials." *J Clin Oncol* 2006; 24(3):419–430.

4. Lu, C, et al. "Chemoradiotherapy with or without AE-941 in stage III non-small cell lung cancer: a randomized phase III trial." *J Natl Cancer Inst* 2010; 102(12):859–865.

5. Prudden, JF. "The treatment of human cancer with agents prepared from bovine cartilage." *J Biol Response Mod* 1985; 4(6):551–584.

6. Romano, CF, et al. "A phase II study of Catrix-S in solid tumors." *J Biol Response Mod* 1985; 4(6):585–589.

7. Puccio, C, et al. "Treatment of metastatic renal cell carcinoma with Catrix (abstract)." *Proc Annu Meet Am Soc Clin Oncol* 1994; 13:A769.

8. Folkers, K, et al. "Survival of cancer patients on therapy with coenzyme Q10." *Biochem Biophys Res Commun* 1993; 192:241–245.

9. Hertz, N, Lister, RE. "Improved survival in patients with end-stage cancer treated with coenzyme Q(10) and other antioxidants: a pilot study." *Anticancer Res* 2010; 30(4):1105–1112.

10. Conklin, KA. "Coenzyme Q10 for prvention of anthracycline-induced cardiotoxicity." *Integr Cancer Ther* 2005; 4(2):110–130.

11. Kunnumakkara, AB, et al. "Curcumin inhibits proliferation, invasion, angiogenesis and metastasis of different cancers through interaction with multiple cell signaling proteins." *Cancer Lett* 2008; 269(2):199–225.

12. Dhillon, et al. "Phase II trial of curcumin in patients with advanced pancreatic cancer." *Clin Cancer Res* 2008; 14(14):4491–4499.

13. Zoltaszek, R, et al. "The biological role of D-glucaric acid and its derivatives: potential use in medicine." *Postepy High Med Dosw* 2008; 62:451–462.

14. Heerdt, AS, et al. "Calcium glucarate as a chemopreventive agent in breast cancer." *Isr J Med Sci* 1995; 31(2–3):101–105.

15. Banerjee, S, et al. "Attentuation of multi-targeted proliferation-linked signaling by 3,3'-diiindolylmethane (DIM): from bench to clinic." *Mutat Res* 2011 (epub).

16. Del Priore, G, et al. "Oral diiindolylmethane (DIM): pilot evaluation of a nonsurgical treatment for cervical dysplasia." *Gynecol Oncol* 2010; 116(3):464–467.

17. Kaegi, E. "Unconventional therapies for cancer: 1. Essiac. The Task Force on Alternative Therapies of the Canadian Breast Cancer Research Initiative." *CMAJ* 1998; 158)7):897–902.

18. Ulbricht, C, et al. "Essiac: systematic review by the natural standard research collaboration." *J Soc Integr Oncol* 2009; 7(2):73–80.

19. Das, UN. "Tumoricidal and anti-angiogenic actions of gamma-linolenic acid and its derivatives." *Curr Pharm Biotechnol* 2006; 7(6):457–466.

20. Kenny, FS, et al. "Gamma linolenic acid with tamoxifen as primary therapy in breast cancer." *Int J Cancer* 2000; 85(5):643–648.

21. Baskshi, A, et al. "Gamma-linolenic acid therapy of human gliomas." *Nutrition* 2003; 19(4):305–309.

22. Kuhn, KS, et al. "Glutamine as indispensable nutrient in oncology: experimental and clinical evidence." *Eur J Nutr* 2010; 49(4):197–210.

23. Savarese, DM, et al. "Prevention of chemotherapy and radiation toxicity with glutamine." *Cancer Treat Rev* 2003; 29(6):501–513.

24. Chen, D, et al. "Tea polyphenols, their biological effects and potential molecular targets." *Histol Histopathol* 2008; 23(4):487–496.

25. Khan, N, et al. "Targeting multiple signaling pathways by green tea polyphenol (-)-epigallocatechin-3-gallate." *Cancer Res* 2006; 66(5): 2500–2505.

26. "USDA Database for Flavonoid Content of Selected Foods." 2003. http://www.nal.usda.gov/fnic/foodcomp/.

27. Larsson, SC, Wolk, A. "Tea consumption and ovarian cancer risk in a population-based cohort." *Arch Intern Med* 2005; 165(22):2683–2686.

28. Zhang, M, et al. "Green tea consumption enhances survival of epithelial ovarian cancer." *Int J Cancer* 2004; 112(3):465–469.

29. Ogunleye, AA, et al. "Green tea consumption and breast cancer risk or recurrence: a meta-analysis." *Breast Cancer Res Treat* 2010; 119(2):477–484.

30. Kurahashi, N, et al. "Green tea consumption and prostate cancer risk in Japanese men: a prospective study." *Am J Epidemiol* 2008; 167(1):71–77.

31. Betuzzi, S, et al. "Chemoprevention of human prostate cancer by oral administration of green tea catechins in volunteers with high-grade prostate intraepithelial neoplasia: a preliminary report from a one-year proof-of-principle study." *Cancer Res* 2006; 66(2):1234–1240.

32. Tsao, AS, et al. "Phase II randomized, placebo-controlled trial of green tea extract in patients with high-risk oral premalignant lesions." *Cancer Prev Res* (Phila Pa) 2009; 2(11):931–941.

33. Shanafelt, TD, et al. "Clinical effects of oral green tea extracts in four patients with low grade B-cell malignancies." *Leuk Res* 2006; 30(6):707–712.

34. Shanafelt, TD, et al. "Phase I trial of daily oral Polyphenon E in patients with asymptomatic Rai stage 0 to II chronic lymphocytic leukemia." *J Clin Oncol* 2009; 27(23):3808–3814.

35. McLarty, J, et al. "Tea polyphenols decrease serum levels of prostate-specific antigen, hepatocyte growth factor, and vascular endothelial growth factor in prostate cancer patients and inhibit production of hepatocyte growth factor and vascular endothelial growth factor in vitro." *Cancer Prev Res* 2009; 2(7):673–682.

36. Pisters, EM, et al. "Phase I trial of oral green tea extract in adult patients with solid tumors." *J Clin Oncol* 2001; 19)6):1830–1838.

37. Aggarwal, BB, Ichikawa, H. "Molecular targets and anticancer potential of indole-3-carbinol and its derivatives." *Cell Cycle* 2005; 4(9); 1201–1215.

38. Naik, R, et al. "A randomized phase-II trial of indole-3-carbinol in the treatment of vulvar intraepithelial neoplasia." *Int J Gynecol Cancer* 2006; 16(2):786–790.

39. Wong, G, et al. "Review: Indole-3-carbinol as a chemoprotective agent in breast and prostate cancer." *In Vivo* 2008; 22(4):441–445.

40. Vucenik, I, Shamsuddin, AM. "Cancer inhibition by inositol hexaphosphonate (IP-6) and inositol: from laboratory to clinic." *J Nutr* 2003; 133 (11 Suppl 1):3778S–3784S.

41. Fox, CH, Eberl, M. "Phytic acid (IP6), novel broad spectrum anti-neoplastic agent: a systematic review." *Complement Ther Med* 2002; 10(4):229–234.

42. Vucenik, I, Shamsuddin, AM. "Protection against cancer by dietary IP6 and inositol." *Nutr Cancer* 2006; 55(2):109–125.

43. Haseen, F, et al. "Is there a benefit from lycopene supplementation in men with prostate cancer? A systematic review." *Prostate Cancer Prostate Dis* 2009; 12(4):325–332.

44. Ansari, MS, Gupta, NP. "Lycopene: a novel drug therapy in hormone refractory metastatic prostate cancer." *Urol Oncol* 2004; 22(5):415–420.

45. Mills, E, et al. "Melatonin in the treatment of cancer: a systematic review of randomized controlled trials and meta-analysis." *J Pineal Res* 2005; 39(4):360–366.

46. Yan, JJ, et al. "Patients with advanced primary hepatocellular carcinoma treated by melatonin and transcatheter arterial chemoembolization: a proespective study." *Hepatobiliary Pancreat Dis Int* 2002; 1(2):183–186.

47. Nahleh, Z, et al. "Melatonin, a promising role in taxane-related neuropathy." *Clin Med Insights Oncol* 2010; 28(4): 35–41.

48. "Modified citrus pectin." *Altern Med Rev* 2000; 5(6):573–575.

49. Lissoni, P, et al. "A study of immunoendocrine strategies with pineal indoles and interleukin-2 to prevent radiotherapy-induced lymphocytopenia in cancer patients." *In Vivo* 2008; 22(3):397–400.

50. Calviello, G, et al. "Antineoplastic effects of n-3 poly-unsaturated fatty acids in combination with drugs and radiotherapy: preventive and therapeutic strategies." *Nutr Cancer* 2009; 61(3): 287–301.

51. Colomer, R, et al. "N-3 fatty acids, cancer and cachexia: a systematic review of the literature." *Br J Nutr* 2007; 97(5):823–831.

52. Ooi, VE, Liu, F. "Immunomodulation and anti-cancer activity of polysaccharide-protein complexes." *Curr Med Chem* 2000; 7(7): 15–29.

53. Kumar, KB, et al. "Inhibition of chemically induced carcinogenesis by drugs used in homeopathic medicine." *Asian Pac J Cancer Prev* 2007; 8(1):98–102.

54. Pathak, S, et al. "Ruta-6 selectively induces cell death in brain cancer cells but proliferation in normal peripheral blood lymphocytes: A novel treatment for human brain cancer." *Int J Oncol* 2003; 23(4):975–982.

55. Frenkel, M. "Homeopathy in cancer care." *Alt Therapies* 2010; 16(3):12–16.

56. Coombs, GF Jr., et al. "Reduction of cancer risk with an oral supplement of selenium." *Biomed Environ Sci* 1997; 10(2–3):227–234.

57. MacFarquhar, JK, et al. "Acute selenium toxicity associated with a dietary supplement." *Arch Intern Med* 2010; 170(3):256–261.

58. Rics, S, Whitehead, SA. "Phytoestrogens and breast cancer—promoters or protectors?" *Endocr Relat Cancer* 2006; 12(4):995–1015.

59. Shu, XO, et al. "Soy food intake and breast cancer survival." *JAMA* 2009; 302(22):2437–2443.

60. Hwang, W, et al. "Soy food consumption and risk of prostate cancer: a meta-analysis of observational studies." *Nutr Cancer* 2009; 61(5):598–606.

61. Kwan, et al. "A phase II trial of a soy beverage for subjects without clinical disease with rising prostate-specific antigen after radical radiation for prostate cancer." *Nutr Cancer* 2010; 62(2):198–207.

62. Shroder, FH. "Randomized, double-blind, placebo-controlled crossover study in men with prostate cancer and rising PSA: effectiveness of a dietary supplement." *Eur Urol* 2005; 48(6):922–930.

63. Yarilin, AA, Belyakov, IM. "Cytokines in the thymus, production and biological effects." *Curr Med Chem* 2004; 11(4):447–464.

64. Constantinou, C, et al. "Vitamin E and cancer: an insight into the anticancer activities of vitamin E and isomers and analogs." *Int J Cancer* 2008; 123(4):739–752.

65. Wada, S. "Chemoprevention of tocotrienols: the mechanism of antiproliferative effects." *Forum Nutr* 2009; 61:204–216.

66. Chang, R. "Bioactive polysaccharides from traditional Chinese medicine herbs as anticancer adjuvants." *J Altern Complement Med* 2002; 8(5):559–565.

67. Fan, TP, et al. "Angiogenesis: from plants to blood vessels." *Trends Pharmacol Sci* 2006; 27(6):297–309.

68. Lin, LZ, et al. "Effect of traditional Chinese medicine in improving quality of life of patients with non-small cell lung cancer in late stage." *Zhongguo Zhong Xi Yi Jie He Za Zhi* 2006; 26(5):389–393. [Chinese.]

69. Wong, R, et al. "Integration of Chinese medicine into supportive cancer care: a modern role for an ancient tradition." *Cancer Treat Rev* 2001; 27(4):235–246.

70. Wang, S, et al. "Molecular basis of traditional Chinese medicine in cancer chemoprevention." *Curr Drug Discov Technol* 2010; 7(1):37–45.

71. Cameron, E, Pauling, L. "Supplemental ascorbate in the supportive treatment of cancer: Prolongation of survival times in terminal human cancer." *Proceeding of the National Academy of Sciences* 1976; 73:3685–3689.

72. Gaziano, JM, et al. "Vitamins E and C in the prevention of prostate and total cancer in men: the Physicians' Health Study II randomized controlled trial." *JAMA* 2009; 301(1):52–62.

73. Creagan, ET, et al. "Failure of high-dose vitamin C (ascorbic acid) therapy to benefit patients with advanced cancer. A controlled trial." *New England J Med* 1979; 301:687–690.

74. Coulter, ID, et al. "Antioxidants vitamin C and vitamin E for the prevention and treatment of cancer." *J Gen Int Med* 2006; 21(7):735–744.

75. Chen, Q, et al. "Pharmacologic ascorbic acid concentrations selectively kill cancer cells: Action as a pro-drug to deliver hydrogen peroxide to tissues." *Proc Natl Acad Sci* 2005; 102:13604–13609.

76. Hoffer, LJ, et al. "Phase I clinical trial of i.v. ascorbic acid in advanced malignancy." *Ann Oncol* 2008; 19(11):1969–1974.

77. Berenson, JR, et al. "A phase I/II study of arsenic trioxide/bortezomib/ascorbic acid combination therapy for the treatment of relapsed or refractory multiple myeloma." *Clin Cancer Res* 2007; 13(6):1762–1768.

78. Garland, CF, et al. "The role of vitamin D in cancer prevention." *Am J Public Health* 2006; 96(2):252–261.

79. Gorham, ED, et al. "Vitamin D and prevention of colorectal cancer." *J Steroid Biochem Mol Biol* 2005; 97(1–2):179–194.

80. Garland, CF, et al. "Vitamin D for cancer prevention: global perspective." *Ann Epidemiol* 2009; 19(7):468–483.

81. Giovanucci, E. "Vitamin D status and cancer incidence and mortality." *Adv Exp Med Biol* 2008; 624:31–42.

82. Beer, TM, Myrthue, A. "Calcitriol in cancer treatment: from the lab to the clinic." *Mol Cancer Ther* 2004; 3(3):373–381.

83. Habu, D, et al. "Role of vitamin K2 in the development of hepatocarcinoma in women with viral cirrhosis of the liver." *JAMA* 2004; 292(3):358–361.

84. Kakizaki, S, et al. "Preventive effects of vitamin K on recurrent disease in patients with hepatocellular carcinoma arising from hepatitis C viral infections." *J Gastroenterol Hepatol* 2007; 22(4):518–522.

85. Calderon, PB, et al. "Potential therapeutic application of vitamin C and K3 in cancer treatment." *Curr Med Chem* 2002; 9(24):2271–2285.

86. Tareen, B, et al. "A 12 week open label, phase I/IIa study using apatone for the treatment of prostate cancer after failed standard therapy." *Int J Med Sci* 2008; 5(2):62–67.

87. Yoshiji, H, et al. "Combination of vitamin K2 and angiogensis-converting enzyme inhibitor ameliorates cumulative recurrence of hepatocellular carcinoma." *J Hepatol* 2009; 51(2):315–321.

Conclusion

1. Azmi, AS, et al. "Proof of concept: network and systems biology approaches aid in the discovery of potent anticancer drug combinations." *Mol Cancer Ther* 2010; 9(12):3137–3144.

2. Peterson, JJ, Novick, SJ. "Nonlinear blending: a useful general concept for

the assessment of combination drug synergy." *J Recept Signal Transduct Res* 2007; 27(2–3):125–146.

CASE STUDIES OF COCKTAIL THERAPY

1. Partin, AW, et al. "Contemporary update of prostate cancer staging nomograms (Partin Tables) for the new millennium." *Urology* 2001; 58(6):843–848.

2. Chen, RC, et al. "Individualizing quality-of-life outcomes reporting: how localized prostate cancer treatments affect patients with different levels of baseline urinary, bowel, and sexual function." *J Clin Oncol* 2009; 27(24):2877–2878.

3. Chaudary, UB, Turner, JS. "Finasteride." *Expert Opin Drug Metab Toxicol* 2010; 6(7):873–881.

4. Yang, Y, et al. "Saw Palmetto induces growth arrest and apoptosis of androgen-dependent prostate cancer LNCaP cells via inactivation of STAT 3 and androgen receptor signaling." *Int J Oncol* 2007; 31(3):593–600.

5. Shenouda, NS, et al. "Phytosterol Pygeum africanum regulates prostate cancer in vitro and in vivo." *Endocrine* 2007; 31(3):72–81.

6. Hsieh, TC, et al. "Prevention and management of prostate cancer using PC-SPES: a scientific perspective." *J Nutr* 2002; 132(11 Suppl):3513S–3517S.

7. Ye, F. "Molecular mechanism of anti-prostate cancer activity of Scutellaria baicalensis extract." *Nutr Cancer* 2007; 57(1):100–110.

8. Aronson, WJ, et al. "Growth inhibitory effect of low fat diet on prostate cancer cells: results of a prospective, randomized dietary intervention trial in men with prostate cancer." *J Urol* 2010; 183(1):345–350.

9. Stupp, R, et al. "Radiotherapy plus concomitant and adjuvant temozolomide for glioblastoma." *New England J Med* 2005; 352(22):987–996.

10. Hegi, ME, et al. "Clinical trial substantiates the predictive value of O-6-methylguanine-DNA methyltransferase promoter methylation in glioblastoma patients treated with temozolomide." *Clin Cancer Res* 2004; 10(6):1871–1874.

11. Kang, KB, et al. "Enhancement of glioblastoma radioresponse by a selective COX-2 inhibitor celecoxib: inhibition of tumor angiogenesis with extensive tumor necrosis." *Int J Radiat Oncol Biol Phys* 2007; 67(3):888–896.

12. Chinnayin, P, et al. "Modulation of radiation response by histone deacetylase inhibition." *Int J Radiat Oncol Biol Phys* 2005; 62(1):223–229.

13. Borbustuc, G, et al. "Levetiracetam enhances p53-mediated MGMT in-

hibition and sensitizes glioblastoma cells to temozolomide." *Neuro Oncol* 2010; 12(9):917–927.

14. Panossian, A, et al. "Rosenroot (Rhodiola rosea): traditional use, chemical composition, pharmacology and clinical efficacy." *Phytomedicine* 2010; 17(7):481–493.

15. Ma, X, et al. "Huperzine A from Huperzia species—an ethnopharmacological review." J *Ethnopharmacol* 2007; 113(1):15–34.

16. Stone, JA, et al. "Mechanisms of action for acupuncture in the oncology setting." *Curr Treat Options Oncol* 2010; 11(3–4):118–127.

17. Velascon, G, et al. "Cannabinoids and gliomas." *Mol Neurobiol* 2007; 36(1):60–67.

18. Seyfried, BT, et al. "Targeting energy metabolism in brain cancer through calorie restriction and the ketogenic diet." *J Cancer Res Ther* 2009; 5 Suppl:S7–15.

19. Grommes, C, et al. "Inhibition of in vivo glioma growth and invasion by peroxisome proliferator-activated receptor gamma agonist treatment." *Mol Pharmacol* 2006; 70(5):1524–1533.

20. Hau, P, et al. "Low-dose chemotherapy in combination with COX-2 inhibitors and PPAR-gamma agonists in recurrent high-grade gliomas—a phase II study." *Oncology* 2007; 73(1–2):21–25.

21. Mastronardi, L, et al. "Tamoxifen as a potential treatment of glioma." *Anticancer Drugs* 1998; 9(7):581–586.

22. Haque, A, et al. "Emerging role of combination of all-trans retinoic acid and interferon-gamma as chemoimmunotherapy in the management of human glioblastoma." *Horm Metab Res* 1992; 24(5):210–213.

23. Baumann, F, et al. "Combined thalidomide and temozolomide treatment in patients with glioblastoma multiforme." *J Neurooncol* 2004; 67(1–2): 191–200.

24. Dale, E, et al. "Chlorimipramine: a novel anticancer agent with a mitochondrial target." *Biochem Biophys Res Commun* 2005; 328(2):623–632.

25. Briceño, E, et al. "Institutional experience with chloroquine as an adjuvant to the therapy for glioblastoma multiforme." *Surg Neurol* 2007; 67(4): 388–391.

26. Martin, V, et al. "Intracellular signaling pathways involved in the cell growth inhibition of glioma cells by melatonin." *Cancer Res* 2006; 66(2): 1081–1088.

27. Lissoni, P, et al. "Increased survival time in brain glioblastomas by a ra-

dioneuroendocrine strategy with radiotherapy plus melatonin compared to radiotherapy alone." *Int J Radiat Oncol Biol Phys* 2007; 68(3):852–857.

28. Trouillas, P, et al. "Redifferentiation therapy in brain tumors: long-lasting complete regression of glioblastomas and an anaplastic astrocytoma under long term1-alpha-hydroxycholecalciferol." *J Neurooncol* 2001; 51(1): 57–66.

29. Das, UN. "Gamma-linolenic acid therapy of human glioma—a review of in vitro, in vivo, and clinical studies." *Med Sci Monit* 2007; 13(7): RA119–131.

30. Yokoyama, S, et al. "Inhibitory effect of epigallocatechin-gallate on brain tumor cell lines in vitro." *Neuro Oncol* 2001; 3(1):22–28.

31. Pyrko, P, et al. "The unfolded protein response regulator GRP78/BiP as a novel target for increasing chemosensitivity in malignant gliomas." *Cancer Res* 2007; 67(20):9809–9816.

32. Ooi, VE, Lui, F. "Immunomodulation and anti-cancer activity of poly-saccharide-protein complexes." *Curr Med Chem* 2000; 7(7):715–729.

33. Mao, XW, et al. "Evaluation of polysaccharopeptide effects against C6 glioma in combination with radiation." *Oncology* 2001; 61(3):243–253.

34.Wakisaka, S, et al. "AUFRAP therapy: combined modality treatment of malignant gliomas with intraarterial infusion of ACNU." *Gan To Kagaku Ryoho* 1988; 15(8 Pt 2):2405–2409.

35. Kang, SG, et al. "Combination celecoxib and temozolomide in C6 rat glioma orthotopic model." *Oncol Rep* 2006; 15(1):7–13.

36. Stockhammer, F, et al. "Continuous low-dose temozolomide and cele-coxib in recurrent glioblastoma." *J Neurooncol* 2010; 100(3):407–415.

37. Padillo, J, et al. "Melatonin and celecoxib improve the outcomes in ham-sters with experimental pancreatic cancer." *J Pineal Res* 2010; 49(3):264–270.

38. Adhami, VM, et al. "Combined inhibitory effects of green tea polyphe-nols and selective cyclooxygenase-2 inhibitors on the growth of human prostate cancer cells both in vitro and in vivo." *Clin Cancer Res* 2007; 13(5):1611–1619.

39. Whitehouse, PA, et al. "Synergistic activity of gamma-linolenic acid and cytotoxic drugs against pancreatic adrenocarcinoma cell lines." *Pancreatology* 2003; 3(5):367–374.

40. Korkmaz, A, et al. "Combination of melatonin and a peroxisome prolif-erator-activated receptor-gamma agonist induces apoptosis in a breast can-cer cell line." *J Pineal Res* 2009; 46(1):115–116.

41. McCarty, MF, et al. "PPAR gamma agonists can be expected to potentiate

the efficacy of metronomic chemotherapy through CD36 up-regulation." *Med Hypotheses* 2008; 70(2):419–423.

42. Wietrzyk, J, et al. "The antitumor effect of lowered doses of cytostatics combined with new analogs of vitamin D in mice." *Anticancer Res* 2007; 27(5A):3387–3398.

43. Caroll, DG. "Use of antidepressants for management of hot flashes." *Pharmacotherapy* 2009; 29(11):1357–1374.

44. Schem, C, Jonat, W. "Expanding role of ovarian suppression/ablation in premenopausal ER-positive breast cancer: issues and opportunities." *Oncology* 2009; 23(1):44, 47.

45. Kenny, FS, et al. "Gamma linolenic acid with tamoxifen as primary therapy in breast cancer. Effect of dietary GLA+/-tamoxifen on the growth, ER expression and fatty acid profile of ER positive human breast cancer xenofrafts." *Int J Cancer* 2001; 92(3):342–347.

46. Walaszek, Z, et al. "Metabolism, uptake, and excretion of a D-glucaric acid salt and its potential use in cancer prevention." *Cancer Detect Prev* 1997; 21(2):178–190.

47. McTiernan, A, et al. "Weight, physical activity, diet, and prognosis in breast and gynecologic cancers." *J Clin Oncol* 2010; 28(26):4074–4080.

48. Giese-Davis, J, et al. "Decrease in depression symptoms is associated with longer survival in patients with metastatic breast cancer: a secondary analysis." *J Clin Oncol* 2011; 29(4):413–420.

Case Studies of Cocktail Therapy

Presented in this section are three distinct cancer cases for which cocktail therapy was successfully implemented. Although they are real-life examples, names have been changed to protect the privacy of the patients. As you will see, the circumstances of each case differ considerably, as do the goals of treatment. Yet, all three scenarios illustrate how cocktail therapy for cancer can be applied efficiently and effectively with the guidance and expertise of a physician. The drugs and supplements mentioned in the following pages should not be used without the supervision of a qualified healthcare professional, and without due consideration of the potential risks, side effects, and interactions.

CASE #1: PROSTATE CANCER THERAPY (WITHOUT CONVENTIONAL TREATMENT)

Joe, a vigorous seventy-one-year-old, had just recently remarried when he was diagnosed with prostate cancer. A routine blood test had showed that his prostate-specific antigen (PSA) level was high, with a reading of 8.2 ng/mL (nanograms per milliliter). For a man of Joe's age, a normal reading is 6.5 ng/mL or less. A subsequent biopsy revealed that his Gleason score (a grade used to measure prostate cancer prognosis) was 6, which indicated about a 25-percent chance that the cancer had spread beyond the prostate.[1]

Joe first consulted a urology specialist, who recommended surgery, followed by a radiation oncologist, who advised brachytherapy. The problem with these treatments, however, is that they pose a high risk of impotence and other side effects,[2] and Joe was adamant in his refusal to compromise life quality. For similar reasons, he declined to undergo hormone therapy, as well as other treatments that would probably render him impotent, but would not necessarily eliminate the prostate cancer.

Then, Joe consulted with me, and I gave him a thorough overview of the risks and benefits of various approaches to treatment. Once I made sure that Joe was clear on his choice to forgo traditional treatments, I proposed a cocktail therapy plan involving off-label drugs, supplements, and dietary modifications.

First, Joe was sequentially treated with off-label drugs, starting with the statin drug simvastatin (Zocor). The COX-2 inhibitor celecoxib (Celebrex) was next, followed by a dihydrotestosterone (DHT) hormone inhibitor called finasteride (Proscar), which is normally used to treat enlarged prostates.[3] These medications are associated with few risks and side effects, and although they are not officially recognized as anti-cancer drugs, their efficacy in cancer treatment is well documented. In general, the three medicines were well tolerated by Joe, but simvastatin caused him to experience some muscle aches. As a result, use of this drug was discontinued.

Dietary supplements were then added to Joe's daily regimen, including vitamin D_3 (5000 IU), lycopene (15 mg), and selenium (200 mcg). He also began taking the herbs Saw Palmetto,[4] *Pygeum africanum*,[5] and a Chinese herbal formula modeled after PC-SPES*[6] that contains the Chinese herb *Scutellaria baicalensis*.[7] One baby aspirin (81 mg per day) was also included in Joe's treatment in order

---

*Between 1997 and 2002, a product called PC-SPES, which is a mixture of extracts from eight herbs based on Traditional Chinese Medicine and backed by over 100 lab and clinical studies, was reported to prohibit prostate cancer and reduce PSA in patients. This product was withdrawn from the US market in 2002 due to concerns about quality control and reported contamination. See Blumenthal, Mark, "The Rise and Fall of PC-SPES: New Generation of Herbal Supplement, Adulterated Product, or New Drug?" *Integrative Cancer Therapy* 2002; 1(3):266–270.

to mitigate the risk of cardiovascular events and deep venous thrombosis, which can be caused by celecoxib and Chinese herbs, respectively. Last but not least, I emphasized the importance of soy, as well as low-fat and high-fiber foods, for prostate cancer management.[8] I advised Joe to lose weight and maintain a rigorous diet, which has been shown to slow the progression of prostate cancer.

Joe's PSA began to decline after following this treatment plan for only two months. After a little more than a year, it was down to a normal reading of 4.3 ng/mL. Joe was elated; his quality of life had not been compromised, and he had lost eighteen pounds. Now, five years since his diagnosis, Joe is healthy, cancer-free, and has a stable PSA.

CASE #2. BRAIN CANCER TREATMENT (WITH CONVENTIONAL TREATMENT)

Unlike breast and prostate cancer, brain cancer—or *glioma*—is relatively uncommon. It is also a deadlier cancer, and in its most common and aggressive form, *glioblastoma multiforme,* the median survival time is only twelve to seventeen months, even when surgery, radiation, and chemotherapy are applied sequentially and intensively. Due in part, perhaps, to the modest therapeutic impact of conventional treatments, and certainly due in part to the fervent effort to discover better treatments, there is a large array of unconventional, integrative, and investigative treatments for glioma. The following case illustrates how a multimodal therapy strategy that includes such treatments can be implemented for brain cancer.

A prominent lawyer at sixty-six years old, John was healthy until experiencing a sudden seizure that led to a diagnosis of glioblastoma multiforme. John immediately sought the opinions of top specialists and decided to undergo surgery, which removed 90 percent of his tumor but left him with slight neurological deficits. He was then scheduled to undergo radiation treatment followed by chemotherapy with temozolomide (Temodar). This type of chemotherapy has been the gold standard for brain cancer management ever since a large European clinical trial reported that it improved the average survival time to 14.6 months, and the two-year survival rate to 26.5 percent.[9]

John's case, however, was different. Not only was he slightly older than the average patient studied in the trial, but his tumor was also more aggressive. Moreover, his tumor had tested positive for the MGMT gene, which allows cancer cells to repair themselves after being damaged by chemotherapy and radiation. This translates into a less than 10-percent chance of surviving eighteen months, even with chemotherapy and radiation, as compared with patients with an inactive MGMT gene, who have a 62-percent chance.[10] In John's case, it would have been unreasonable to try temozolomide chemotherapy until it failed, as he might have been too weakened and incapacitated to endure further treatment. Therefore, I suggested that we try to enhance the effectiveness of the conventional treatment—radiation and chemotherapy—with cocktail therapy.

During the radiation phase of treatment, which also included low doses of chemotherapy, John began taking the COX-2 inhibitor celecoxib to boost the cancer cells' radiosensitivity.[11] Valproic acid (Depakote) and phenylbutyrate (Buphenyl), which act as an epigenetic therapy,[12] were also considered, but John could not tolerate valproic acid. Instead, he was put on levetiracetam (Keppra), another antiepileptic drug that has been shown to enhance MGMT gene silencing and increase tumor sensitivity to temozolomide chemotherapy.[13] To counter negative side effects of radiation, I recommended the herbs Rhodiola for fatigue[14] and Huperzia serrata for memory.[15]

The next phase of John's treatment was regular-dose temozolomide chemotherapy cycles. He continued to feel fatigued and experience significant nausea, causing him to lose weight. In order to reduce his nausea and improve his overall quality of life, John began to receive acupuncture regularly.[16] He also started taking the cannabis derivative tetrahydrocannabinol (THC), or Marinol, to boost his appetite and prevent further weight loss. (THC has been reported to work effectively against glioma,[17] which was another reason for prescribing the drug.) John began to meet with a nutritional counselor and follow a modified ketogenic diet, which is a low-carb and high-fat regimen that is often used to treat epilepsy and may improve brain cancer outcomes.[18] The diet is not an easy one to follow, but with the help of a customized computer program to generate recipes, a liquid ketogenic formula called Ketocal, the medical food caprylidene (Axona), and some discipline, John was able to stick to the diet.

Six weeks into chemotherapy, John became increasingly unable to tolerate temozolomide, though his scans remained stable. As a result, he was switched to metronomic (low-dose and less toxic) chemotherapy and put on the drug pioglitazone (Actos), a PPAR gamma modifier, at 30 mg per day.[19] He also continued to take 200 mg of celecoxib daily. This combination is a modified version of a regimen used in a German study that implemented the cocktail strategy to treat glioma.[20] Other anti-glioma drug combinations that have been reported as potentially beneficial were considered as well, such as tamoxifen (Nolavadex),[21] all-trans retinoic acid (ATRA) or Retin-A,[22] and thalidomide (Thaldomid).[23] Ultimately, this combination was not attempted due to concerns about possible toxicity.

So, at this point, John's treatment regimen included the following medications:

- Celecoxib (Celebrex), 200 mg twice a day

- Levetiracetam (Keppra), 500 mg twice a day

- Pioglitazone (Actos), 30 mg once a day

- Temozolomide, 50 mg/m^2 per day

- THC (Marinol), 5 mg three times a day

This regimen was tolerated quite well, and after three weeks, two more off-label drugs were added: chlorimipramine (Anafranil), an antidepressant, and the antimalarial drug chloroquine (Aralen). Chlorimipramine has shown to directly kill glioma cancer cells,[24] while chloroquine can more than double the survival time of patients with glioblastoma multiforme.[25] Thus, John added 50 mg of chlorimipramine (taken at bedtime) to his daily regimen, as well as 250 mg of chloroquine phosphate.

At the same time, the following dietary supplements were incorporated into John's treatment program:

- Gamma-linolenic acid (GLA), 240 mg twice a day

- Green tea extract (standardized to 50-percent EGCG), 500 mg twice a day

- Huperzia serrata (standardized to 200 mcg huperzine A per capsule), 2 capsules per day

- Melatonin, 20 mg at bedtime

- PSP or PSK (*Coriolus* mushroom extract), 3 g per day

- *Rhodiola rosea* (standardized to 3-percent rosavin), 200 mg twice a day

- Vitamin D3, 5000 IU once a day

Most of the supplements on the list above have been extensively studied as potential cancer treatments, are not associated with any serious toxic effects, and have been shown to be effective for brain cancer. For instance, at very low concentrations, melatonin has decreased the growth of glioma by as much as 70 percent in only seventy-two hours, according to animal studies.[26] In human-based studies, a combination of melatonin and radiation has improved survival for glioma patients.[27]

A number of studies have also indicated that vitamin D and its analogs may inhibit glioma cells. A French study, for example, found that 1-alpha-hydroxycholecalcifeol (alfacalcidol), a form of vitamin D, increased the four-year survival rate of glioblastoma patients by 20 percent.[28] Results of numerous studies on gamma-linolenic acid and glioma have been encouraging as well.[29]

Although there have not been any trials of green tea catechins specifically for brain cancer treatment, there is some laboratory evidence that they can suppress glioma cells.[30] Moreover, EGCG may improve the effectiveness of temozolomide chemotherapy for brain cancer.[31]

Finally, there is a breadth of medical literature supporting the use of PSP and PSK for improving the quality of life and survival time of patients who have various types of solid tumors.[32] PSP has been found to sensitize glioma cells to radiation,[33] and PSK may be used with chemotherapy and radiation against glioma.[34]

The combination of agents used for John's cancer has been reported to work synergistically, which is another reason why these specific substances were chosen. Some of these synergistic (and potentially synergistic) combinations are:

- Celecoxib (Celebrex) and temozolomide chemotherapy[35, 36]

- Celecoxib and melatonin[37]

- COX-2 inhibitors and EGCG[38]

- GLA and chemotherapy[39]

- PPAR gamma agonists and melatonin[40]

- PPAR gamma agonists and metronomic chemotherapy[41]

- Vitamin D and low-dose chemotherapy[42]

Although there are plenty of other effective supplements and drugs that John could have been prescribed, his quality of life may have been negatively affected if additional substances were included in his daily regimen—he was already taking over two dozen pills per day. Therefore, he continued to take only the drugs and supplements already mentioned, while maintaining a modified ketogenic diet and visiting an acupuncturist each week to help his lack of appetite and fatigue. John also started to see a psychotherapist and explore energy-enhancing exercises such as Qi-gong. As of the publication of this book, John is still living.

CASE #3: HIGH-RISK BREAST CANCER PREVENTION

Eva, a forty-year-old executive, was generally in good health despite being slightly overweight, and having high cholesterol and borderline-high blood sugar. Quite unexpectedly, Eva was diagnosed with a hormone-sensitive, high-risk breast cancer with lymph node involvement. She had a lumpectomy, a standard procedure, followed by intensive chemotherapy and radiation to prevent the cancer from returning. Afterwards, Eva was prescribed tamoxifen (40 mg per day), an anti-estrogen drug frequently used to treat breast cancer and inhibit its recurrence. However, the medication caused adverse side effects, including hot flashes, sleeping problems, and depression. In addition, as a residual side effect of chemotherapy, Eva experienced "brain fog," or cognitive impairment characterized by poor memory and the inability to think clearly. These side effects added to Eva's stress level, but her oncologist insisted that tamoxifen was her only option.

Subsequently, Eva consulted with me and learned the possible ways to deal with tamoxifen side effects, and even avoid its use. Her hot flashes could be simply treated with a supplement like vitamin E (2000 IU per day) or, alternatively, SSRI antidepressants such as venlafaxine (Effexor),[43] which would potentially also help her depression. (The dosage would be titrated, or adjusted, until the optimal result was achieved.) Acupuncture was another option for Eva, since it has been shown to reduce hot flashes, alleviate stress, and promote weight control. And if Eva continued to experience adverse side effects from tamoxifen, LHRH agonists (a type of hormone therapy) like goserelin (Zoladex) could be used instead to medically suppress her ovaries, thereby lowering her risk of cancer recurrence.[44] Surgical removal of the ovaries was yet another treatment option; this would reduce the amount of estrogen in Eva's body. The tamoxifen regimen would then be replaced with an aromatase inhibitor, a class of drugs used to decrease estrogen levels in women who have breast cancer.

I also informed Eva of various off-label drugs that may reduce the risk of breast cancer recurrence and could be used in place of tamoxifen. These include cholesterol-lowering statin drugs, anti-diabetic agents such as metformin, and bisphosphonates, which may also improve survival. Eva could begin a regimen of each medication gradually, taking the next drug only after determining that the previous one had not caused any negative side effects.

If Eva opted to continue using tamoxifen, though, I recommended some supplements to provide further benefits. For example, gamma-linolenic acid, or GLA, may work synergistically with tamoxifen to more effectively fight breast cancer.[45] Additionally, supplements such as indole-3-carbinol (I3C), diindolylmethane (DIM), calcium D-glucarate, and vitamin D_3 may positively influence estrogen metabolism.[46]

Finally, quality of life is an important issue in cancer treatment and management, and for this, Eva was presented with a number of options. For brain fog resulting from chemotherapy, she could take gingko biloba or phosphatidylserine, two dietary supplements that are associated with memory improvement. Weight reduction is also beneficial for overall physical and mental well-being (not to mention breast cancer prevention), so I recommended that Eva follow a low-fat and low-sugar diet in order to lose some weight. Diets low in fat and sugar, moreover, are linked to a lower breast cancer risk.[47] Lastly, I advised Eva to see a therapist to deal with her depression, and consider joining a support group to improve her mood and overall outlook on life. A healthy mental state is correlated with better immunity, which, of course, would improve Eva's chances of cancer survival.[48]

It has been over five years since Eva first consulted me and, as of the publication of this book, she remains cancer-free. She has not been on tamoxifen since reaching menopause; now she takes the aromatase inhibitor letrozole (2.5 mg per day), which is not causing her any adverse side effects. Eva's diet is now healthier than ever and, as a result, she has lost a significant amount of weight. Better yet, she is no longer depressed, so her quality of life has dramatically improved. Eva's case serves as a model for a multidimensional and more holistic approach to cancer treatment that touches upon a patient's physical, psychological, and emotional health.

CONCLUSION

Although these cases have different circumstances and levels of complexity, all three demonstrate how cocktail therapy can be effectively and safely implemented. This multidimensional approach creates more personalized and, often, more comprehensive treatment plans than those typically offered by conventional therapy. Anti-cancer cocktail therapy can improve not only quality of life for patients as they undergo treatment, but also their survival.

About the Author

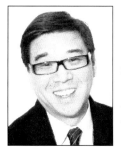

Dr. Raymond Chang received both his BA and MD degrees from Brown University, and subsequently completed postdoctoral training at Yale and Cornell hospitals. He then joined the staff of Memorial Sloan-Kettering Cancer Center, where he served for ten years until 1997. He has been on the faculty of the Weill Cornell Medical College since 1986.

Dr. Chang is acknowledged as one of the pioneers of complementary and alternative medicine in the US, especially in the field of oncology. He founded the nonprofit Institute of East-West Medicine in 1997 towards integrating Eastern and Western approaches to medicine, and currently directs the world's largest database project on anti-cancer Asian herbs. Dr. Chang has lectured widely on herbal medicine, integrative oncology, and alternative medicine over the past three decades. He has served on editorial and advisory committees of various academic journals and presided over international conferences for East-West approaches to cancer, as well as non-Western medical traditions.

Dr. Chang is currently in private practice in New York City.

Index

OTHER SQUAREONE TITLES OF INTEREST

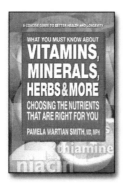

WHAT YOU MUST KNOW ABOUT
VITAMINS, MINERALS, HERBS & MORE
Choosing the Nutrients That Are Right for You
Pamela Wartian Smith, MD, MPH

Almost 75 percent of health and longevity is based on lifestyle, environment, and nutrition. Yet even if you follow a healthful diet, you probably don't get all the nutrients you need to prevent disease. In *What You Must Know About Vitamins, Minerals, Herbs & More,* Dr. Pamela Smith explains how you can maintain health through the use of nutrients.

Part One of this easy-to-use guide discusses the individual nutrients necessary for good health. Part Two offers personalized nutritional programs for people with a wide variety of health concerns. People without prior medical problems can look to Part Three for their supplementation plans. Whether you want to maintain good health or you are trying to overcome a medical condition, *What You Must Know About Vitamins, Minerals, Herbs & More* can help you make the best choices for the health and well-being of you and your family.

$15.95 US • 448 pages • 6 x 9-inch quality paperback • ISBN 978-0-7570-0233-5

NATURAL MEDICINE,
OPTIMAL WELLNESS
The Patient's Guide to Health and Healing
Jonathan V. Wright, MD, and Alan R. Gaby, MD

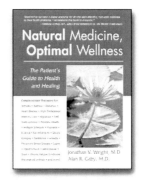

Imagine having holistic physicians at your fingertips to answer your medical questions. With *Natural Medicine, Optimal Wellness,* you do. For each condition, you'll sit in on a consultation between Dr. Jonathan Wright and a patient seeking advice. By the conclusion of each visit, you'll have a complete understanding of why Dr. Wright prescribes particular natural treatments. Then, in a separate commentary, Dr. Alan Gaby follows up with an analysis of the scientific evidence behind the treatments discussed, enabling you to make informed decisions about your health.

If you wish to receive the best of care from the best of physicians, *Natural Medicine, Optimal Wellness* is the natural choice for your personal library of health and wellness books.

$21.95 US • 400 pages • 8.5 x 11-inch quality paperback • ISBN 978-1-890612-50-4

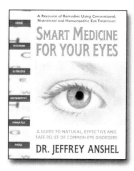

SMART MEDICINE FOR YOUR EYES

A Guide to Natural, Effective, and Safe Relief of Common Eye Disorders

Jeffrey Anshel, OD

Trouble can start with headaches and blurred vision, or simply with redness and tearing. Certainly, going to an eye-care professional is essential, but to be part of the solution, you must be informed. That's why *Smart Medicine for Your Eyes* was written. Here is an A-to-Z guide to the most common eye disorders and their treatments, using both conventional and alternative care.

This easy-to-understand book is divided into three parts. Part One provides a simple overview of how the eyes work, and introduces methods of treatment from acupuncture to nutrition. Part Two is a comprehensive directory to child and adult eye disorders and their various treatment options. Finally, Part Three guides you in using the procedures suggested in Part Two. *Smart Medicine for Your Eyes* is a reliable source of information that you will turn to time and again to protect the greatest of your possessions—your eyes.

$19.95 US • 424 pages • 7.5 x 9-inch quality paperback • ISBN 978-0-7570-0301-1

THE YIN & YANG OF CANCER

Breakthroughs from the East and the West

Bernard Chan, MD, and Georges M. Halpern, MD, PhD

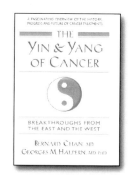

Although Eastern and Western doctors have the same objectives in the fight against cancer, their methods of treatment are worlds apart. *The Yin & Yang of Cancer* bridges the information gap between these two approaches. The authors begin with a clear history of how traditional Chinese and Western medicines evolved, and how they have interacted with each other. They then provide a detailed discussion of the Chinese use of medicinal mushrooms, which could add further weapons to our own cancer-fighting arsenal.

$15.95 US • 160 pages • 6 x 9-inch quality paperback • ISBN 978-0-7570-0207-6

For more information about our books, visit our website at www.squareonepublishers.com